FINDING PEACE OF MIND THROUGH SELF-DEFENSE

GERONIMO T. WATSON

Printed in the United States of America
ISBN: Softcover   979-8-89518-126-3
           eBook   979-8-89518-127-0

Republished by: WP Lighthouse
Publication Date: 06/06/2018

To order copies of this book, contact:
WP Lighthouse
Phone: 1-888-668-2459
support@wplighthouse.com
www.wplighthouse.com

Contents

Here's Your Package

May I personally thank you for your decision to subscribe to the *Anshin Self Defence and Streetwise Awareness Course.* This course has been developed especially for you after many years of "trial and error" techniques, some of which have been improved and some of which had to be abandoned.

The Law:

"Section 3 of the Criminal Law Act 1967 states that a person may use force that is reasonable and necessary in the circumstance." It also states *"such a person must be able to justify their actions in a court of law"*

We will explain this legal terminology later in the course under the heading of **Streetwise**.

The techniques and real life scenarios that you are about to learn are not fictitious, on the contrary, all the following information has been taken from real situations that either myself or my fellow karate ka (karate practitioners) have been involved in over many years.

Although the techniques have been perfected in the dojo, they have been "practised" on the street with "Mr. Joe Public".

Once again may I thank you for purchasing our system of self-defence and as my personal hero Bruce Lee once said, the best style of a martial art is;

"The art of fighting without fighting"

心
の
平
静

REMEMBER:

Prevention is better than the Cure

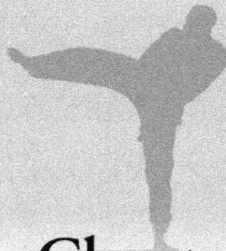

Chapter 1
Introduction of Instructor

Before I begin with the introduction to both your course, and myself, I would like to apologise if the grammar and the punctuation are not of a literary genius. Writing has never been one of my strengths as I have a habit of "telling it as it is"!

My name is Graham Summerfield and I am a fully qualified professional karate and self defence instructor. I have been teaching and training in karate for nearly 30 years and currently hold the "rank" of 5th Degree Black Belt in Wado Ryu Karate Do. As well as teaching the traditional syllabus we also train in other forms such as BJJ, Judo, Boxing, Dim Mak and joint manipulation. Although now retired from competition, I have represented Shindo-Kai many times in the UK, I am also a coach with the Shindo Kai Karate Association and regularly coach our fighters in competitions on the EKF circuit.

I am fully insured with Professional Indemnity, DBS checked and qualified to coach with the "E.K.F." (English Karate Federation), who answers to both the Government and The Sports Council. We are also 1st aid trained.

At present my company, Anshin Karate & Self Defence (Anshin meaning "peace of mind" in Japanese) teaches self-defence at Barnsley and Wakefield Colleges, plus karate in many of Barnsley's Primary schools as well as our evening classes. We have also been contracted to teach self-defence as part of the P.E. curriculum in many of the secondary schools within the Barnsley, Wakefield, Sheffield, Leeds, Rotherham and Doncaster areas, these include;

BARNSLEY SCHOOLS:

Darton High School
Dearne High School
Willowgarth High School
Priory School & Sports College
Penistone Grammar School
Royston High School
Kingstone High School
St. Michaels Catholic & C of
E High School Foulstone High
School
Holgate School & Sports College
Wombwell High School
The Elmhirst School
Edward Sheerian School

SHEFFIELD SCHOOLS:

Bradfield Comprehensive School
Hinde House School
Chaucer School
Ecclesfield School
East Hill Special Needs School
Meadowhead School
High Storrs School
Notre Dame High School

ROTHERHAM SCHOOLS:

Rawmarsh Community School
& Sports College

WAKEFIELD SCHOOLS:

Knottingley High School
St. Thomas A. Beckett
Crofton High School
Hemsworth Arts & Community
College
St. Wilfrids Catholic High School
Cathedral School
Rodillian School
The Kings High School
Kettlethorpe High School
Horbury High School
Outwood Grange College

LEEDS SCHOOLS:

Horsforth School
Benton Park School
Farnley Park High School
Temple Moor School
Wetherby High School
John Smeaton Community High
School
Corpus Christi Catholic College
Primrose High School

DONCASTER SCHOOLS:

Don Valley High School

The reason behind publishing this course is simple. Over the last few years, teachers and adults have asked me to teach them the same fundamental tactics to increase their awareness and street sense.

There are simply not enough hours in the day for me to coach everyone face to face, so the obvious answer was for me to create our very first self-defence manual.

✳✳✳

What does self-defence mean?

In short it is every human beings right to defend themselves with the up most force when faced with a dangerous or threatening situation.

3 easy steps you can take are;

x.   trust your instincts, if something doesn't feel right, then more then likely it isn't
xi. look for the danger signs early
xii. be confident physically and mentally

3 vital strike areas;

i.   eyes
ii. throat
iii. groin

When people talk about self-defence, everyone immediately thinks of an 8 stone woman throwing a 15 stone man over her shoulder and stamping on his groin. When in reality many situations can be avoided by using common sense tactics and talking your way out of a situation. Learning to be positive and assertive are a must. Self-defence also includes communication skills, streetwise tactics and positive body posture. There are many techniques we can use before combat. Not all attackers are strangers, 4 out of 10 men who attack women are already known to the victim, even friends and family members have been convicted of physical and sexual abuse.

The following course is designed to teach even the most timid person to evade conflict and deal with physical confrontation should it arise. On this course you will learn that everyone has vulnerable areas, especially men, and that all would be victims have the weapons within their own bodies to use against these areas.

"An assault is an act of power over another person"

"The basic rule of self-defence is to reverse that power thereby taking control of the situation"

20 years ago the police's stance on such attacks was that the victim should not resist, as fighting back may increase the chances of sustaining an injury.

However, the FBI conducted a 10 year study involving over 1.5 million rape victims, their conclusions were:

"Injuries sustained by women who fought back were no different from those who did not. It was a myth that the risk of injury, mutilation or even death was increased by resistance. In fact it was found that women who resisted by using some form of self-defence, actually doubled their chances of escape".

Women were seen and indeed saw themselves as victims. This perception alone could be interpreted by a potential assailant as an invitation to attack. Even today there are many "rape crisis centres", "victim support groups", and "police rape units" which are set up to help victims deal with the trauma of physical and sexual attacks.

However there are all too few specialist education centres who focus entirely on self-defence so that you may be prepared and armed against potential and actual situations.

The art of self-defence is not just taught to fight off men, sometimes a woman may attack another woman. Even though rape or sexual assault may not be on the agenda, the same principles of self-defence apply.

Fighting is a last resort – only to be used if your life depends upon it. You are highly likely to sustain some type of injury if you fight, but you must weigh up the cost of injury against the costs incurred if you **do not** fight back.

Today if someone is being attacked (man or woman) in a very busy street, surrounded by numerous passers by, it is highly likely that you will still be alone and no one will come to help. There was an experiment conducted on a famous breakfast television show some years ago, where a lady acted as though she had been involved in a RTA (road traffic accident). She lay motionless in the gutter of the road, car after car swerved to miss her and pedestrian after pedestrian walked straight by. The reason; no one wants to get involved. In today's society everyone just wants to live in their own little bubble and not move out of their comfort zone.

To summarise – **do not expect help from anyone!**

One of the 1ˢᵗ rules of self-defence is to get your **reactions** on the same level as your opponent's **actions**. In other words if your attacker is angry you have to become just as angry as him. FACT: attackers are cowards, they always go for the weakest victim who they know will not fight back or resist their advances. Body language and fences will be covered later on in the course.

Self-defence is not just about physical manoeuvres, 70% is mental preparation, not being in the wrong place at the wrong time, the knowledge of how to behave when faced with danger. Being able to "buy" time and "distract" the attacker so that you can make your escape.

The human brain is the best computer ever made and controls many functions, but women's are very different from men's. We all have a Human brain, a Mammalian brain and a Reptilian brain.

The human brain in a woman is larger that of a man, this is why women can "multi-task". When face with danger the women will instinctively run away to keep the body from harms way. Where as the man, (due to our stone-age ancestors) would rather fight than run. It has not changed for thousands of years. For example, if a girl was about to fight in the playground, but she decided to run instead, nothing really would be said. However if a boy was faced with the same situation and he ran away, he would be branded a chicken, or a coward. Right or wrong this is the way it is.

The mammalian brain is the same size in both sexes. This controls involuntary responses such as blinking, sneezing, shivering etc.

The reptilian brain is smaller in a woman than that of a man. Stone-age man scenario again, men would rather fight........................... IDIOTS!

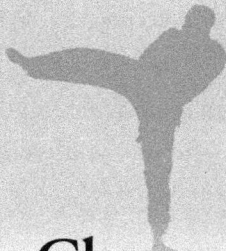

Chapter 2
Your body's own natural weapons

E veryone has the same number of natural weapons, I know this because we are all human. Not given the fact that some of the population have had amputations, we all have 5 weapons; 2 arms, 2 legs, 1 head. These weapons can then be sub divided into more definitive areas.

Arms – shoulders, elbows, fists, fingers

Legs – thighs, knees, feet

Head – forehead, teeth (biting however is a last resort as we do not know if the assailant suffers from any contaminating diseases, HIV, Aids, Hepatitis A, B, or C, Chlamydia, or other STI.

Arms

Shoulders make incredible weapons if used correctly, rugby players and American football players can testify to this.

There are 4 main types of elbow strike, and again when delivered correctly will literally flatten an opponent, these are;

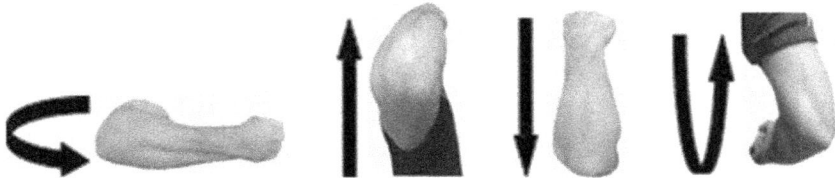

E i)   E ii)   E iii)   E iv)

E i)   Front elbow strike - imagine grabbing the back of an attackers head and driving your forearm and elbow directly to the face in an out to in motion

E ii)   Upwards elbow strike – this normally is used when an attacker comes towards you and you then strike him upwards to either his nose or his chin

E iii)   Dropping elbow strike – if the attacker is smaller than you or if the attacker has bent over (maybe you have just struck his groin) you will then drop your elbow either onto the top of his head, his nose or his collar bones (clavicle), the back of his neck, or his spinal column

E iv)   Backwards elbow strike – specifically designed if you are attacked from behind, drive that elbow into his face or his chest or his groin

Firstly, we shall dismiss the myth that the hand can be made into only 1 fist, in actual fact there are 4 areas of the fist we can utilise:

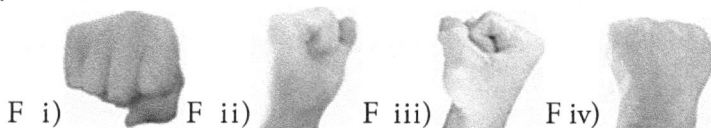

F i)   F ii)   F iii)   F iv)

F i)   front of the fist (normal punch using the 3rd knuckles in line to hit an object)

F ii)   bottom of the fist (padded area below the little finger executed in a downward motion)

F iii)   top of the fist (when all fingers are clenched, this is the area on top utilising the index finger and thumb)

F iv)   back of the fist (area of the hand between 3rd knuckles and wrist – meta carpals)

Fingers can be utilised in all sorts of ways. We could poke eyes, grab flesh, scratch skin, or the ultimate – grab and twist the genitals.

Legs

Be careful, thighs can be used as a weapon, alternatively we all know how much it hurts if we get a "dead leg".

Knees and feet are self-explanatory so we shall not waist time going over the obvious.

Head

Head butting is well known as a form of attack so need for discussion here. Biting?! Please read above.

Chapter 3
Striking Points & Fences

Striking Points

Atemi Waza (striking points of the human body)

We shall now discover that fingers and hands are much more of a weapon than mere fists, below is a diagram of the human form with numbers corresponding to strike areas. Please refer to this when reading on. We shall work from the top of the head to feet explaining, "Which strike goes where".

N.B. Some of these striking points will hit nerve endings resulting in violent pain for the attacker, temporary paralysis and even death. Please use extreme caution when practising these techniques as we accept no responsibility for injuries sustained by "your volunteer". I, like many instructors within our industry, have been training and teaching these sort of techniques for many years, and, although we know the damage they may cause, we always use the up most control when demonstrating to avoid unnecessary accidents.

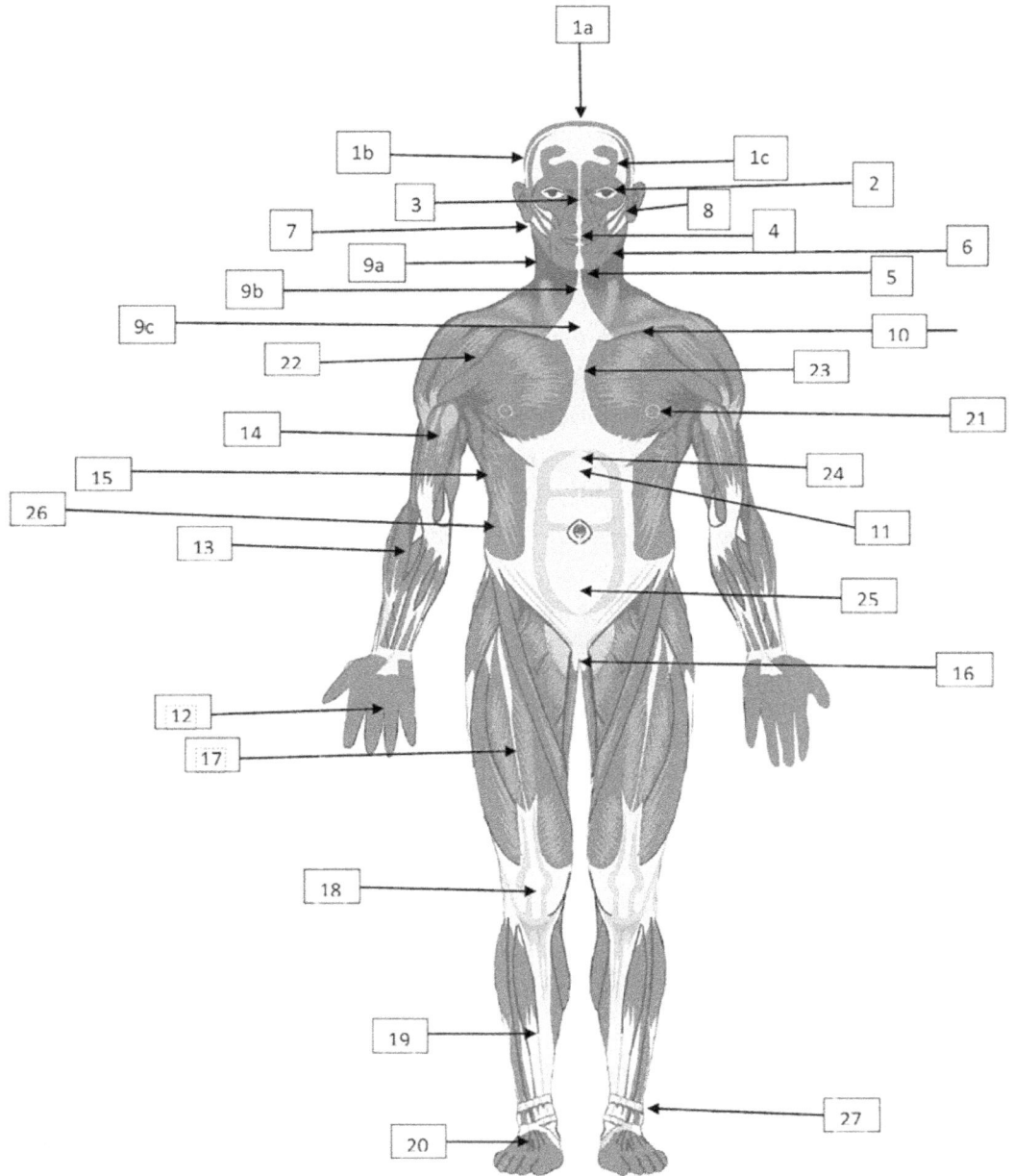

1. a) Top of The Head

Delivering a blow to this part of the head with a "hammer fist strike" (bottom area of the fist – atemi waza – F ii), will do one of two things. It will either give the attacker a massive headache, or in a severe case, it will induce a brain aneurysm causing the brain to bleed uncontrollably. If the latter occurs there is only a 2.5% chance of survival without any side effects.

Case study –

My wife suffers from high blood pressure relating to polycystic kidney disease. In 2005 she suffered a brain aneurysm whilst doing the weekly shop, after being scanned it was decided to operate. The doctors wrapped the burst artery in a copper coil which is still in place to this day. Prior to this we were briefed upon the procedure. "10% of people who suffer this type of trauma do not make it to hospital, if they do 5% do not survive the operation. If they are really lucky and do survive the operation, there is a 50-50 chance that they will endure some kind of brain damage. Hence the 2.5%.

b) Back of the Head

Hitting here with any form of strike will cause pain, paralysis or even death

c) Side of Head – temple

Striking the temple would again result in a "knockout" blow, using either of the strikes below;

i.   using the back of the fist (F iv) in a roundhouse motion

ii.   using bottom of the fist (F ii) padded area below little finger executed in a roundhouse motion

Hitting here or indeed anywhere on the skull would result in the same type of injury

Please only use these techniques if your life depends upon it!

The Law:

"Section 3 of the Criminal Law Act 1967 states that *a person may use force that is reasonable and necessary in the circumstance."* It also states *"such a person must be able to justify their actions in a court of law"*

2. Eyes

To gouge someone in the eyes is extremely painful for the recipient. We all know how painful it can be even if we accidentally poke ourselves in the eye, or even have an insect fly into it.

Please only use this technique if your life depends upon it!

The Law:

"Section 3 of the Criminal Law Act 1967 states that *a person may use force that is reasonable and necessary in the circumstance."* It also states *"such a person must be able to justify their actions in a court of law"*

Could you justify in a court of law blinding someone? Let us imagine for 1 second that you were in the rape position, this huge smelly guy is on the top you, he takes one hand away from your wrist or neck to unzip his trousers and you manage to gouge his eyes out. Remember the only thing these people react to is pain, you cannot reason or plead with them...... they are criminals.

No court in the land would convict you of doing something that was reasonable and necessary in the circumstance. However if you escaped from your assailant and then went back and shot the guy, then you would most definitely be convicted of murder. We will cover this in more detail in Chapter 4.

3. Bridge of the nose

Anyone who has broken their nose is all too aware of the pain that is caused, headaches, black eyes etc. Speaking from experience and 2 very painful operations (rhinoplasty), I can tell you the pain is excruciating.

There are 3 small lateral bones in the nose (I know this because I don't have them anymore) which if bumped or broken cause severe pain to the victim.

Using the fist there are 2 basic strikes which can be performed,

i. using the normal fist (F i)

ii. using the back of the fist (F iv) in a vertical motion

4. Between the bottom of the nose and the upper lip

Below the nose is also a striking point. Between the nostrils is a piece of gristle called the septum, if this were to be struck either with a normal punch or with the heal of the hand; the consequences would be very severe. The septum would be pushed up into the 3 lateral bones in the nose, which would in turn be pushed up into the front of the brain causing death.

Please only use this technique if your life depends upon it!

The Law:

"Section 3 of the Criminal Law Act 1967 states that *a person may use force that is reasonable and necessary in the circumstance."* It also states *"such a person must be able to justify their actions in a court of law"*

Also under the nose on the top gum can also be used as a deterrent. The slightest pressure on this area will cause the attacker to back off and think again.

5. Chin

A strong punch, kick, or strike to the chin is used more than any other area on the body to cause "knockout".

6. Jaw/Mandible

The jaw can be used as a "knockout" area in the same way as the chin, but on the jaw we can use 2 different types of fist,

i. The back of the fist (F iv) in a roundhouse motion

ii. The bottom of the fist (F ii) padded area below little finger executed in a roundhouse motion

7. Under the Ears

Striking someone here would not result in major trauma but would assist in sending a warning to the person that you are not going to be such a push over. There is a small cavity behind the ear - just at the back of the ear lobe - between the back of the lower jaw and the base of the skull. Normally we would use a one knuckle fist for maximum pain, but just to prove a point, use your index or forefinger and push firstly in horizontally, then upwards at 45°. Your opponent will raise from the soles of their feet onto their toes without you even touching their legs.

8. Ears

Ears are not automatically thought of as a striking point but when utilised correctly may become extremely painful. If someone came to grab you or if they succeed in grabbing you, this is one of many techniques which are unbelievably effective. Imagine your attacker has his arms on your lapels or worse, around your throat. Simply cup your hands to form a concave shape, then slam these cupped hands into the assailant's ears. The resulting injury would be that of burst ear drums and probably bleeding from the upper skull. The reason being is that as you slam your cupped hands into his ears the air that is present in your hands is pushed at great speed and pressure into his ear cavity, thus bursting his ear drums

9. Neck and Throat

These two areas can be extremely painful and even fatal if hit correctly.

In the neck there are a number of "pipes"; nerves, tendons, ligaments, veins and arteries. To strike these vulnerable areas is a last resort.

a) To the Neck

We could use either a punch, "karate chop" or other strike could result in the recipient being disorientated or worse.

b) To the Throat

Options are more varied, although I prefer the open hand technique rather than the fist. This open hand technique is most commonly used after "putting up a fence" (these will be explained more in detail later). The striking hand is spread wide and then close the fingers, palm flat with just the thumb out on its own. The hand is then thrust into the throat using the skin line from the tip of the index finger to tip of the thumb.

c) To the base of the throat

Between the collar bones and the sternum we all have a small indentation. At this junction we could thrust our forefinger in as deep as possible, then bend the finger and drive it down behind the sternum. Once the finger has reached its maximum depth, if the attacker has not let go of you by this time (more fool him), pull sharply outwards towards your own body.

In extreme cases this movement could pull the collar bones (clavicle) and the sternum clear out of the chest cavity obviously resulting in death!

Please only use this technique if your life depends upon it!

The Law:

"Section 3 of the Criminal Law Act 1967 states that *a person may use force that is reasonable and necessary in the circumstance."* It also states *"such a person must be able to justify their actions in a court of law"*

10. Collar Bones

The clavicle or collar bones like any other bones in the human body are essentially hollow, bone marrow and fat being the major elements that fill the bones. Anyone who has broken a collarbone will know the excruciating pain that is felt. Even pinching the bones between index finger and thumb can cause discomfort.

The strikes to be used here are much the same as in other situations;

   i.   using bottom of the fist (F ii) padded area below little finger executed in a vertical motion

   ii.   the old "karate chop" using the blade of the hand

11. Solar Plexus

This area is primarily used to wind someone. The solar plexus is a muscle located at the bottom of the sternum.

To find the solar plexus on yourself simply draw your fingers down your sternum until you find the end, then place 2 fingers side by side and use the 3rd finger of the other hand to push. You will feel discomfort, and, if you push hard you may even wind yourself.

The reason behind this is simple. The solar plexus is located directly beneath the diaphragm, which in turn is located directly beneath the lungs. When the solar plexus is struck or depressed, this pushes the diaphragm upwards and exhales all the air from you lungs. Literally you will not be able to catch your breath.

12. Hands

Hands and especially fingers and thumbs are easily hurt, fingers by being bent backwards, and thumbs by pushing the thumb print downwards into itself.

13. Forearm

The forearm contains two bones, radius and ulna. Generally where a major bone exists there is also along side it, a major nerve. Close to the radial and median bones are the radial and median nerves, if these are pressed or struck correctly "pins and needles" run the length of the entire arm and the arm is rendered useless for up to 10 minutes, sometime even longer. Although it does take practice to find and administer pressure at the correct point, once mastered there is no defence.

The strikes used can be either;

i. using bottom of the fist (F ii) padded area below little finger executed in a vertical motion

ii. the old "karate chop" using the blade of the hand

We shall briefly try to explain the nerves location. Hold the arm out straight as if performing a normal punch with the knuckles horizontal, run your fingers from the outside of the elbow to the inside of the elbow, then back to the top of this line. Use the "2 fingered rule" again to come down towards the fist and then use 1 finger to come inside towards the forearm muscle, push or hit. As was discussed previously this is not easy but once mastered is extremely effective.

14. Upper Arm

The radial nerve continues up the arm and can be located on the inside of the bicep muscle, hit this and the same discomfort is felt. A strike to the armpit will render the assailant harmless due to the large nerve endings causing temporary paralysis to the whole arm.

15. Back

Hitting the spinal column is extremely painful and can result in serious injury or worse. As too can hitting the kidneys, too hard and renal failure will follow. The sciatic nerve is also located in this region which if struck can cause searing pain to the victim.

Please only use this technique if your life depends upon it!

The Law:

"Section 3 of the Criminal Law Act 1967 states that a person may use force that is reasonable and necessary in the circumstance." It also states *"such a person must be able to justify their actions in a court of law"*

16. Groin

Not much to be said here, except ladies, if you are ever in a position where you are frightened for your life, do not be afraid to what ever is necessary to this area. Punching and hitting is fine, but for example if you were to be grabbed from behind and hitting is not an option, then grab, squeeze, tear etc. I think you get the message!

17. Thigh

As briefly mentioned earlier the thigh can be really painful if hit correctly. This is the science bit;

We all have four muscles in our thigh (quadriceps) and these are mainly working the front of the leg so we may bend and squat etc. Although "dead legging" is painful it is exaggerated when received on the outside of the thigh. Why? Well in everyday use the muscles are not in contact with the thigh bone (femur), they are suspended or attached to the bone with tendons.

If we get "dead legged" the muscles are pressed inwards and touch the bone, bone as we know contain many properties, one of which is calcium. The pain comes from the calcium touching the muscle.

Top Tip

If you do suffer from a "dead leg or arm" please do not rub the site. Rubbing causes friction, which generates heat, this heat then accelerates the chemical transfer from bone to muscle. If this transfer is prolonged it has been known for part of the muscle to turn to bone, this is irreversible.

Instead of rubbing, try to walk it off, or scream if you want, BUT DO NOT RUB!

18. Knees

Knees are wonderful joints, but very fragile. Hinges, ligaments, cartilage, fluid are all present in the knee joint. The knee is only capable of one type of movement. If possible, when confronted with potential danger, kick or stamp on the knee so it bends backwards like the leg of a bird. Alternatively kick it sideways to dislocate the knee cap.

19. Shins

Shins are made of skin, blood and bone, in that order. There are no muscles or fat present, this is why it hurts so much when you receive a blow. Should your attacker come from behind and grab you or choke you, one of the effective ways to dismiss him is to drive your heel into his shins, this plus the "5 point plan" (which we cover in chokes & strangles) will ensure your escape.

20. Instep

Simple, if you are being grabbed from behind as above, drive your stiletto heal straight through his foot into the concrete - he will let go!

21. Nipples

The nipples are very sensitive areas which if hit with any form of strike will cause the tiny blood vessels behind the nipple to burst resulting in extreme pain.

22. Front of Shoulder

By using fists or fingers to penetrate behind the shoulder muscle put pressure on nerve endings which may disable the attackers arm for enough time for you to make your escape.

23. Heart

No need for explanations here, hit too hard will result in death.

Please only use this technique if your life depends upon it!

The Law:

"Section 3 of the Criminal Law Act 1967 states that *a person may use force that is reasonable and necessary in the circumstance."* It also states *"such a person must be able to justify their actions in a court of law"*

24. Diaphragm

This muscle controls the movement (inhalation and exhalation) of the lungs, which if disrupted by a punch or a kick will cause the victim to be "winded".

25. Abdomen below navel

A strike here could cause, shock, internal bleeding and unconsciousness.

26. Floating Ribs

The floating ribs are named such due to them not being attached to anything, unlike the rest of the ribs which are attached to sternum and the spine. Fractured ribs can cause punctured lungs and main organ failure.

27. Lower Leg

Both the calf and the Achilles tendon are located in the lower leg, which if struck correctly will bring any sized opponent to their knees.

Fences

Fences are designed to keep a safe distance between you and a potential attacker. Remember talking distance is arms length, keeping your arm straight and in a locked position up against the attackers chest.

There are 3 fences which are very effective;

i.   Staggered fence

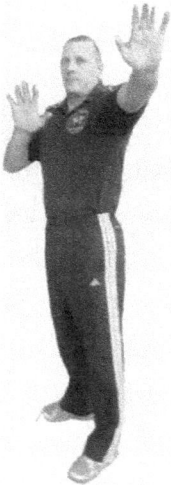

ii. Submissive fence

iii. Psychological fence

Staggered fence

The staggered fence is exactly how it sounds, one arm is extended outwards in a locked position against the attacker's chest, whilst the other is in a bent position ready to strike if required. IMPORTANT – all fences are performed with hands spread open. DO NOT MAKE FISTS, psychologically, open hands = peace, while fists = aggression. If someone came up to you and you immediately showed a staggered fence with fists clenched, that would send a signal to the attacker that you were about to hit him. In self-defence as mentioned before, fighting back is a last resort. We must try and neutralise the situation without combat and with open hands meaning peace we can do just that, plus most important of all, open hands gives us the added advantage of surprise. The attacker thinks we will not strike, when in reality if the attacker breaks our fences down (reduces talking distance by bending our front arm) our back arm or hand is ready to deliver a life changing blow.

Submissive fence

The submissive fence is exactly how it sounds. We submit or surrender. Just as in western movies or police shows, the first thing a victim will do when threatened with a gun or a knife is raise both arms and hands up with palms facing the attacker. Again the attacker thinks we are cowardly or afraid because our hands are spread open, when in actual fact we are ready to strike with either hand or even both if the attacker comes any closer.

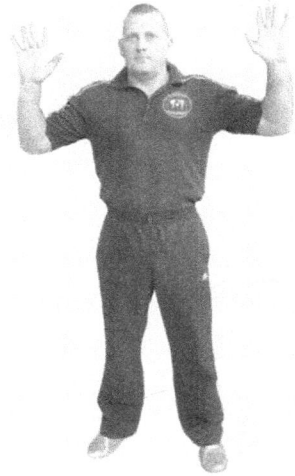

Psychological fence

This type of fence has no physical traits about it whatsoever. This fence is always about bluffing, learning to get your reactions on the same level as your opponent's actions. I am not a big advocate of fowl language, but in the right circumstance and at the right time nothing is more powerful than a few expletives.

For example if you were using a staggered fence and someone came close to you, which would work best;

"Back off" said in a really quiet timid voice

or

"F***ING BACK OFF" shouted in a really aggressive tone

REMEMBER: these people who do these things are cowards, they only pick on the weakest victim. They do not want to get hurt themselves. Be confident.

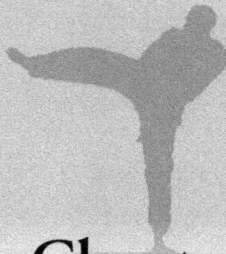

Chapter 4
Awareness, Body Language, Becoming Streetwise

This section of the manual is very, very, very long. Please bear with me while I try to explain all there is to being prepared for an attack. There is a lot of information to take in during this section, so it may be advisable to read this chapter a few times. Although fighting is sometimes a necessity, in most situations combat can be avoided by trusting your instincts and looking for danger signs early. Remember **Prevention** is better than the **Cure**

Awareness

How do we know if we are being followed? We all have a sixth sense, we all know when something is not right. How many times have you being followed, intentionally or otherwise, and you instinctively turn around to see who it is. Sometimes when we are getting closer to home, we drop our guard, this makes us even more vulnerable to an attack.

Looking in shop windows or car windows for reflections or shadows on street corners will decrease the odds of you becoming yet another victim.

There is one problem here, I have just made you subconsciously paranoid. The last thing I want is for you to become a quivering wreck! So, to bring things into context, how do you establish that you are indeed being followed?

Scenario:

You are walking home alone late in the evening and you hear footsteps behind you, they get closer and closer and closer, until eventually you panic, turn around, gouge the guy's eyes out and spatter his groin all over the inside of his trousers. Will this poor man sue you, damned sure he will.........I would!

Little did you know that this man has recently moved into your cul-de-sac. He has been married for 20 years, has 3 children and is looking forward to the weekend watching his youngest play football. He is returning home after a few games of snooker with his mates, 6 or 7 glasses of his favourite tipple, kebab with chilli sauce, most of which is down his shirt, minding his own business. YOU PANIC AND RUIN BOTH YOUR LIVES!

So what do I do?

You must qualify or prove that this person is following you, so here is what you do.

Once you have heard footsteps behind you, you look for traffic and cross over the road. The guy, if he means you harm, cannot grab you from across the road. Keep looking behind you every so often, if he then crosses over as well, this is still no time for you to panic, he may live on this side of the street. Keep crossing over 3, 4 or even 5 times to establish that you are indeed being followed. If he keeps crossing also, then alarm bells begin to sound in your brain, you must come up with a plan, and quickly.

Question?

You are going to be attacked. Would you rather be attacked from behind or from the front?

Answer

From the front every time. From behind you are obviously disadvantaged, whereas from the front you are in a position to attack the vital areas and even use a weapon (not a gun or a knife, but something found in your pocket or handbag, this is covered in **Streetwise**)

Body Language

To have positive body language could mean the difference between rape and not, mugged or not, or even between life and death.

Positive body language will deter an attacker and pass him over to someone less confident than yourself. I know this sounds mean, but we cannot protect every one, I wish we could. The best we can do is to limit the number of attacks happening in today's society.

Some people are naturally confident, while some are really shy and introvert. Confidence only comes from knowledge, if for example you were to sit an exam without knowing what the subject was, naturally you would be nervous and apprehensive. On the other hand, if you were to sit an exam and you knew all the answers before starting, how great and confident would you feel?

Self-defence is no different. People who study martial arts for years generally never get involved in trouble on the street. Why? Well learning to block, kick, and punch correctly, together with learning the real "nasty" stuff such as Dim Mak (death point touching) and nerve fighting, equips the individual to such a high standard, that they become so confident that they know how to fight, that they never have to fight.

To put things in plain English, body language can be broken down into 2 pretend scenarios;

i. The first woman is walking down a street with her back hunched, head down, eyes looking towards the pavement, talking really small fast steps.

ii. The second woman is walking some distance behind her being exactly the opposite. She is walking really tall with her back straight, head and eyes are looking forward having eye contact with people walking in the other direction. Her strides are long and purposeful.

Who is going to make the easiest target?

Becoming streetwise

This is also a really long section so please bear with me. I hope you have a good imagination because a lot of this information is going to put into scenario form based on real life situations. At the end of in the course is a small quiz, the answers will be on the following page from the quiz but please have a go without the answers and see if you really are "streetwise".

70% of self-defence is mental preparation, knowing how to behave when in danger, "buying time", distracting the attacker enabling you to either escape or render the attacker harmless. Fighting is always the last option, never confront unless your life depends upon it. There are 4 main ways to deal with an attack;

i. Yell, make noise, and attract attention. (Yell or shout, do not scream. Shouting opens the diaphragm and helps release adrenalin from the thyroid gland to the main muscle groups helping you to either fight harder or run faster. Screaming constricts the throat so has the opposite effect)

ii. Escape or try to escape

iii. Outside intervention – help from a third party (highly unlikely)

iv. Physical resistance – fighting back

Act upon your instincts, they are your first warning system. Do not think about your attacker or try to "work him out". If escape is impossible, act immediately. The longer your assailant is in control, the worse your situation will get.

If you are not attacked immediately, then be aggressive with your body language and use verbal skills to escape.

DO NOT try to clam him down – he wants to be powerful and in control. Trying to calm him down will probably make you look weak and this in turn may fuel his anger.

DO NOT believe anything he may say or promise – criminals lie!

DO NOT make deals with these people – criminals lie!

Expect no mercy from an attacker, by lying down and submitting simply tells the attacker that he has chosen the easiest target. If someone threatens you with a weapon, but does not immediately show it, there is a 50/50 chance that he is bluffing.

GOLDEN RULE: if you can, run away. You will not get hurt if you are ½ mile away.

We have quoted the law in numerous stages along our journey;

The Law:

"Section 3 of the Criminal Law Act 1967 states that *a person may use force that is reasonable and necessary in the circumstance."* It also states *"such a person must be able to justify their actions in a court of law"*

Now let's break this mumbo jumbo down into something we all can understand.

Someone puts his hands around your waist in a busy pub and asks you your name. If your reaction was to gouge his eyes out and knee his groin, this would be an over reaction and one that would get the police involved.

If someone in town was holding a knife to your throat and told you that they were going to sexually assault you and your reaction was the same, the police should say that the force exerted was in line with the threat of rape or even murder.

If someone rapes you with the threat of a knife being present and they get convicted of rape, they can expect to serve 15 years in prison – out in 7-8 years.

If someone rapes you without the threat of a knife being present and they get convicted of rape, they can expect to serve just 7 years – out in 3-4 years to do it again!!!!!!

To make things simple there are 3 types of behaviour which require 3 different types of action:

1. <u>Nuisances</u>

None threatening behaviour, for example pinching your bottom in a crowded pub or putting their hand on your waist telling you that you are gorgeous.

<u>Action</u>

Simple verbal put downs, dirty looks, moving their hands away from your waist and saying a firm "NO". If you were to over react in this situation and slap the person, shout at him and generally embarrass him in front of all his friends, this could lead to a much more serious situation later. This is not to say that you should allow his behaviour to go unpunished, let them know in non-abusive way that you will not stand for it. Remember drink and drugs play a large part in our society and people can turn violent very quickly, they cannot think responsibly and act very rashly without any thought of the consequences.

2. <u>Situations leading up to a possible attack</u>

Threatening behaviour, stood in front of you stopping you going past them, asking you to go somewhere with them, placing a hand on your shoulder.

<u>Action</u>

Again do not over react, but be aware of the danger that could quickly arise from the situation. Be even more firm and assertive, be confident in your voice and posture. You must tell them you not interested, leave you alone and back off. Tell them that you will shout if they do not move, tell them your partner is waiting for you, or even that you will call the police. Try to make them aware of the consequences of their actions. It may be that they have too much to drink and your actions so far will make them see sense and they will back off. You may get loads of verbal abuse but at least you have defused the situation and are walking away unscathed.

3. <u>Actual bodily confrontation</u>

Someone has grabbed you from behind, or in front. Someone has lunged towards you and makes a grab or swing at you. This is the most serious situation and one that you will need actual self-defence techniques to get you out of harms way.

<u>Action</u>

In a fight, the person who is hit first has a 90% chance of losing the fight. If you are hit first your chances of fighting the attacker off will have diminished considerably. A full on fight will last no more than 5-10 seconds, at this point one person has clearly lost the fight. Stay alert, focused and in control. Maybe a weapon is shown and at that point it would be too life threatening to physically do anything, waiting for a better chance to escape would be safer.

FINDING PEACE OF MIND THROUGH SELF-DEFENSE

Rape is an act of power. Each year in Britain over 200,000 women report an attack

I often get asked the question,

"What happens if I kill someone whilst defending myself". I quote the law –

"Section 3 of the Criminal Law Act 1967 states that a person may use force that is reasonable and necessary in the circumstance." It also states *"such a person must be able to justify their actions in a court of law"*

There are 2 main sentences in this country for killing someone, Murder and Manslaughter.

For those of you that do not know the difference, I will try to explain. Please forgive my rough interpretation, I am no barrister or judge.

Manslaughter is the unlawful killing of a human being without malice aforethought. In other words it was an accident, you did not mean to kill, but nevertheless you did kill someone.

Murder is the unlawful premeditated killing of a human being by another. In other words you planned the killing, you meant to kill.

If convicted of any of the above offences you can expect a custodial sentence. Although circumstances may dictate individual cases the general "rule of thumb" is this –

If convicted of manslaughter the maximum sentence normally given is 15 years, good behaviour etc. will see that sentence reduced to ½ this, i.e. 7-8 years.

If convicted of murder the maximum sentence normally given is 25 years, again good behaviour etc. will see that sentence reduced to ½ this, i.e. 12-13 years.

31

Now let's look at 2 different but quite similar scenarios:

i.   You are in nightclub at around 2am, a guy has been "giving you the eye" for a while but has not approached you. Your friends leave to get something to eat, while you go to the toilet. Upon leaving the club, the guy jumps you, takes you around the back of the building and puts you in the rape position. You are obviously scared out of your wits, this smelly big guy is looking down on you telling you what he is going to do. He then takes one hand away from your wrists to unzip his trousers, you have one hand free, and you immediately start scratching about looking for a weapon. A brick or bottle literally comes to hand and you strike the rapist on the head, he then falls off you unconscious. You run to the nearest police station and report the incident.

Will you get prosecuted in a court of law? Definitely not. You were doing something that was **reasonable** and **necessary** in the circumstance.

ii.   Same scenario with you coming out of the club and being abducted. He again has you in the rape position, takes one hand away from your wrist, you find an object and strike him with it. The guy falls away and you run. You get about 50 meters away and a "light bulb" shines on the top of your head, you think "that b**tard was going to rape me". So you walk back where you find the man still lying unconscious, bleeding from his wound. You are so angry that you look around and you find a piece of paving slab, you then pick it up and slam it down onto the mans face.

Will you get prosecuted in a court of law? You bet.

In the first scenario you will not be held accountable, no court in the land will find you guilty of any offence. BUT, there is always "SODS LAW". For those of you who do not what sods law is, it`s simple; if you do a good deed like helping an old woman across the road, the odds are that no one will witness it. But the moment you do something wrong there will always be a witness or a CCTV in the vicinity.

I, along with my colleagues have worked in women's groups where our students were actual victims of rape. I can tell you it really did upset me to think that some scumbag had totally ruined these ladies lives, they looked at us as though we had just been scraped from the soles of their shoes.

Rape could not only ruin your life.....it lasts for life.

So back to the original question -

"What happens if I kill someone whilst defending myself".

I cannot tell you what to do, only you will know how you would react in such a nasty situation. The one thing I can say is that you will not get convicted by using self defence as in scenario

i.   outline above. How ever if SODS LAW does come into the equation and you are found guilty of manslaughter, you will serve 7-8 years if well behaved.

Decision:- 7-8 years or LIFE sentence!..............as I said before, it's your choice, all I can do is give you the information and let you act upon it.

One of the things that happens when people come under intense pressure is our natural bodies "fight or flight" response. This is when adrenaline is pumped around your body to make you ready to run from danger or to fight the danger off. It is a response that has derived from stone-age times when the dangers of every day living were considerable.

Your heart rate will increase, your strength will increase, awareness is heightened and blood is pumped around your body to the major muscles readying them for action. This is called adrenaline rush. Unfortunately, for every reaction, there is an equal and opposite reaction.

So after an encounter when the heart has returned to its normal rate, the strength subsides, awareness goes back to normal and blood pressure has decreased, you may feel heavy in the legs. You may get an upset stomach, or feel sick inside. This is known as adrenaline dump. The speed in which the adrenaline returns to the thyroid gland will determine the severity of the dump and in turn how sick you feel.

Adrenaline is a natural chemical made by the human body, it is a brilliant pain killer but it also has "super human" properties. Many stories have been published about mere mortal people doing extra ordinary things, for example a woman in the USA lifted a car up into the air so she could free her trapped child.........amazing!

Less than 1% of all rapists are convicted.

If all fails and you do become another victim, do not give up, keep working, we need to lock these scumbags away. I know, easy for me to say, I am a guy, but nevertheless I have a family including a wife and a daughter. I have taught the same techniques to them with the hope that they never have to use them, but fore warned is fore armed!

There are things you can do whether you escape or not to help bring this "thing" to justice:

▶ Look for any distinguishing marks such as birth marks, tattoos etc.

▶ Take notice of their accent

▶ Remember the colour of their skin and hair, what style its in, long, short, curly, straight etc.

▶ Any details of clothing

All these things will assist the police in building a profile of the attacker and hopefully catching him.

If an assault has occurred, do not go home, do not wash your self. Call the emergency services and get to the police station as soon as possible. D.N.A. samples are becoming increasingly more important in catching criminals. May be you scratched your assailant and still have his skin under your nails, may be he kissed your neck and his saliva is still present, and if the unthinkable happened and he did rape you, his D.N.A. would still be there. Even particles of clothing have been known to be contributing factors in the catching of criminals.

One really important point I should make. The police play a vital role in our society and do their best to keep us safe. The reality is though however, that today, we live in such a politically correct world that the rapists, muggers, paedophiles, murderers, robbers and all other criminals are given representation by the authorities even if they cannot afford one themselves. It is the defending solicitor's job to "get their clients off" regardless whether they actually think their client is guilty or not. Therefore if you are attacked and report the incident would you;

a. Make a statement as soon as possible, or

b. Wait for a solicitor to speak to you and help you with the statement

b. Every time. Why? You are not a fully qualified solicitor, if you make a statement on your own, the defending lawyer will twist things around, (that's his job) and make it look as though it were your fault that you were attacked, thereby freeing his client.

Always wait for a solicitor to come, you can ask for a female one if you like. Put your statement in legal terminology that the courts will understand, and hopefully get a conviction.

When I was a child my mother told me a phrase which only made sense to me in later years

"Better to be 10 minutes late than dead on time"

She still says it to me now if I am driving too fast, you know what mums are like!

Always take the route home that is well lit, well populated if possible. NEVER travel through desolate areas, through woodland or down alley ways. Taking short cuts could be your downfall. Being 10 minutes late for your dinner or meeting someone is not worth the risk.

If you do walk down the street and you see an alley coming up on your left hand side, stop, look for traffic and cross over the road before you reach the entrance to the alley.

How to enjoy a night out safely.

We all like to go out from time to time, with friends, or to social events such as weddings or christenings. When we are sober and have our wits about us, we feel safe and in control, but there is always danger lurking around every corner. There are many drugs and substances around today, a lot of which can be slipped into a glass or a bottle.

Rohypnol (flunitrazepam) is commonly known as the date rape drug. It can vary in size and colour but generally it is around 5mm in diameter, the effects however are exactly the same regardless of appearance. The drug is a paralysing drug. The drug, if slipped into your glass will start to work in around 90 seconds, it initially will make you feel light headed or dizzy, and it will start to work on other parts of your body. After a couple of minutes you will get paralysis in your legs and you will collapse, the rest of your body will follow suit and after 10 minutes you will be totally paralysed and unconsciousness will ensue. It is odourless, colourless and tasteless, (you cannot smell it, see it or taste it), you will not know its there.

Following various victims' accounts of Rohypnol, one of the worst things about this drug is that every fibre in your body is paralysed. The guy has you in the rape position (remember rape is an act of power, the sex part of rape is a by product. This scumbag wants to look into your eyes while he is doing the unthinkable, this is why 9 times out of 10 the rape position is the same as the missionary position, i.e. the woman is on her back looking up and the guy is laid on top of her). While you are in this position, you cannot feel anything.

You may think that is a good thing, but also be aware that whilst you cannot move any of your limbs, the drug has paralysed your whole body. In other words you cannot scream or shout for help, but most of all you cannot blink, close your eyes or look away. You are witnessing first hand yourself being raped and there is nothing you can do about it.

PLEASE, PLEASE, PLEASE, never let your drink out of your sight. Keep your thumbs over bottles and hand over glasses. Always see your drink being poured or prepared and take it every where you go, even to the toilet, put it on top of the toilet, do what you have to and bring the drink out with you. If a good looking guy who you fancy offers to buy you a drink, not a problem, go to the bar with him and see your drink being prepared – lager/beer - poured, bottle - opened or cocktail – stirred/shake

Date rape drugs come in many forms but all do the same damage.

Q. If some one dropped something into your glass on a Saturday night at 7 pm, would you know?

A. Yes probably. The pub is relatively empty, quite, there is no music booming out, and most importantly, you are sober.

Alternatively

Q. If some one dropped something into your glass on a Saturday night at 11.30 pm, would you know?

A. Probably not. The pub is heaving with people bumping into you all the time, the music is really loud, and, yes, you have guessed it, you are absolutely drunk!

Some sick people now have starting using Rohypnol for recreation, no not in that way, but watching people make a fool of themselves. It has been reported recently that some young men have been throwing handful's of Rohypnol into the air and waiting for it to fall into either men's or women's drinks. They have no intention of raping them, but they get a kick out of watching the victim fall on the floor paralysed.

Remember Rohypnol is just like any other drug, overdose can KILL!

People get drunk, some more frequently than others, but we have all been there. There are two types of drunken people, please be patient while I try to explain.

Person No1, drink, drink, drink. Eventually have had enough and plateau – this means they get really giddy and silly, then all they want to do is go to sleep.

Person No.2, drink, drink, drink. Eventually they have had enough and they too plateau – instead of being silly and wanting to go to bed, what do this idiots want to do?.................FIGHT!

Some pubs charge to get in, sometimes just a small fee of a few pounds. They want you to stay at their place and spend your money behind THEIR bar. This is an ideal scenario, remember, you cannot take your drinks onto the dance floor for health and safety reasons (broken glass etc), you also do not leave your drink alone. If you have a best friend that you have known since birth do you trust them? NO, unless they have been on an awareness course like this one. You want to go to the toilet and your best friend offers to look after your drink for you, you say thanks but I will take it with me. The reason for this is that if you leave your drink with them, there is a good chance that a song will come on which they want to dance to and they get up leave all the drinks, including yours, and go to dance. These drinks are asking to be spiked. You come back from the toilet 10 minutes later (we all know how long the queues are in the ladies don't we?) and everyone is sat back at your table. How do you know if your drink is safe?

This pub, which you have paid to get into, has some awesome tunes but they are all separated by rubbish ones. Working on the golden rule that if you leave your drink alone its "dead", imagine this. A song comes on that you all want to dance to, what do you do?:

Leave your drink

Or

"Finish it"

Yep, good answer, "Finish it". It would be a real waste of money keep leaving your drink.

However, think about this. How many dances could you fit into a 1 hour period? 10, 20, 30?

We will be really conservative and say 10. Lets think; 10 dances = 10 drinks in 60 minutes.

You come out of the pub into the fresh air and wham, you are going to be totally drunk.

PLEASE think about what you are doing.

Formaldehyde is basically known as "embalming fluid". For those of you who still do not know what is I will try to explain;

This chemical dates back thousands of years to ancient Egyptian times when mummification was at its peak. It is still used very much in the same way today. When you die, firstly cause of death has to be ascertained. A post mortem is carried out to ensure no foul play has taken place, then the body is sent to a "chapel of rest" to await either burial or cremation. As soon as the body dies, its starts to rot from the inside out. We all have many chemicals inside our bodies including hydrochloric acid which is used to break our food down. Sometimes it takes as long as 2 weeks for our bodies to be laid to rest, just imagine the smell and decomposition that would take place in that period.

Formaldehyde is pumped into the corpse and slows down this process keeping the corpse in "state" so that when the relatives say their final farewells, their dear ones just look as if they are sleeping and not like something out of Michael Jackson's "Thriller".

As usual in today's sick society, someone somewhere always finds a use for things that we dismiss as harmless. Formaldehyde is no different. In its raw state, or when its is in its liquid form it really smells foul, but unfortunately it is just like methylated spirits and evaporates really quickly. It has the same traits as Rohypnol when it is dry, i.e. it is odourless, colourless and tasteless, (you cannot smell it, see it or taste it). The scumbags do not put it in your drink, they have started to dip the filters of cigarettes in it. The chemical evaporates immediately, then they offer you one. The effects of formaldehyde are different from Rohypnol in that instead of paralysing you, the drug is hallucinogenic. It makes you hallucinate, you will see things coming out of the walls that you wouldn't believe.

So the major rule here is the same as when you were small children and your parents said; "Do not accept sweets from strangers". The same is true when you get older, do not except things from strangers unless you are absolutely sure they have not been tampered with.

Burglaries

To have someone break into your house is a most traumatic experience, but to have someone break in whilst you are asleep is the ultimate scare.

Q. What would you do if someone broke into your house at 2 am while all the family were asleep?

Possible answers:

A. Run down stairs to confront the burglar, what if he is not alone and there is a gang of criminals

A. Barricade you and your dearest in a bedroom and call the police, this unfortunately would give the burglar enough time to steal your possessions.

If you were to confront the burglar and startle him, two things happen;

a.   You have put him on his guard because he did not expect you to be there and he will do anything to escape

b.   He now may wish to hurt you or possibly kill you because unless they are wearing a mask, you can recognise them.

Case study

A few years ago in 2002 a farmer named Tony Martin confronted 2 travellers who were trespassing on his land, thinking they were out to steal from him, he chased them away and fired his shot gun. One of the travellers unfortunately died from the gun shot wound and Tony Martin found himself in prison for a long time at her Majesty's pleasure.

In today's society you cannot physically stop someone from stealing your valuables. Why? Well in a few instances when the victim has tried to stop the burglar, the burglar has been injured and then accused the victim of assaulting him. The victim is then held to account and the burglar gets off without even a caution..........IT HAPPENS!

Common sense advice – if someone breaks into your house and you feel brave enough to confront him, the end result will be that either you or the burglar will sustain some type of physical injury.

Lets imagine for a moment that the case goes to court because you hurt the burglar, what would you say when questioned?

"I hit him because he was steal my 50 inch plasma T.V." wrong answer, you will go to prison.

What you should say is;

"I have a family upstairs asleep (a wife, son, daughter, baby, it doesn't matter), this guy came into my house threatening me, I was afraid for myself

and my family, so I did what any human being should do, and that was to get this guy out of my house. We got into a fight and that is how the guy got hurt.

It is the burglar's word against yours. Remember the law:

"Section 3 of the Criminal Law Act 1967 states that *a person may use force that is reasonable and necessary in the circumstance."* It also states *"such a person must be able to justify their actions in a court of law"*

Taxis and Buses

Doesn't mean a lot, does it? Catching taxi's or buses wrongly could ruin your evening.

Taxis

There are 2 things we must look for on a taxi cab to ensure it is a legal taxi.

i.   Licence badge on the outside, this can vary in colour from city to city, for example in Sheffield it is yellow and in Salford it is red. Not that this matters, it does the same job, on the licence plate you will find the drivers licence number, the registration number of the vehicle and how many seats it has for transportation.

ii.   I.D. badge on the inside. This is generally a credit card sized badge that is displayed either on the rear view mirror or from one of the vents, it must be on display at all times. On it you will find the same information as on the licence plate plus the driver's passport photo and his name.

You must not get into a taxi, unless it has these two things present.

Here is another top tip:

If you are travelling alone in a cab where would you sit? At the front? At the back? Where about in the back?

Always sit at the back near the kerb opposite the driver. As soon as you get in check for the child locks, make sure they are not on. It is a fact that some drivers have young families who they ferry to and from school, then go to work at night, sometimes they leave them on by accident. Once you are in the taxi, close the door, then immediately open it again just to check. The driver will not say anything, but in case he does…. LIE. Just say something like "sorry mate I didn't think I had shut the door properly".

There is a very good reason for doing this drill. Thousands of taxis are caught everyday without any drama, but once is all it takes:

Case study.

A few years ago in London, a lady caught what she thought was a taxi after an evening out. The cab drove straight passed her house, she tried calling 999 but her mobile phone was dead, she tried opening the door but the child locks were on. Unfortunately she was sat directly behind the driver. I know what some of you are thinking right about now, why didn't she hit him, hmmmm, not a good idea when the cab is travelling at 40 mph to knock the driver unconscious. The driver stopped in a woodland area, put his hands between his legs and pushed his seat all the way back trapping her legs. Calmly he opened his door, opened her door and raped her!

NEVER, NEVER, NEVER sit behind the driver

A good practice to try to get into is to pre-book your taxi. If you know you are going out on a Saturday night at 8 pm, then book it at 12 noon the same day. Do not leave it too late as most will have been taken by then. At the same time that you are booking the outward journey also book the return journey, it's so much easier. Taxi ranks these days can be dangerous places, people pushing and shoving, jumping the queue. I personally have seen more trouble erupt in these places than anywhere else, so please use your common sense.

Think about this true analogy;

3 pm on a Wednesday afternoon – 1 little old lady and 30 cabs to choose from

Midnight on a Saturday night – 30 drunken people and 1 cab which comes every 15 minutes or so.

<u>Buses</u>

The rule on catching buses is more or less the same. If you are catching your last bus home late at night never sit at the back, always sit near the driver.

Scenario:

You have just got on the last bus home and you are alone. 2 to 3 stops later 2 youths get on who are absolutely off their face either on drink or drugs. They walk straight passed you to the back of the bus, giving you some twisted compliment such as "look at the legs on her". Moments later they start with the abuse, do you fell scared, you should. Now you are face with a dilemma, do you get off the bus?

NO...........eventually the bus will either run out of diesel or it will go back to the depot for the night....wrong answer.

YES YOU DO get off the bus. But where do you get off, (you do not have to wait for a bus stop, have a quick word with the driver and he should let you off where ever you want), do you get off before where you live or after where you live? Please refer to the sketch below for your answer;

a.   Before where you live

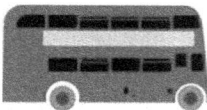

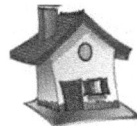

you live here

Direction of travel of the bus

WRONG: you get off before where you live, start running as fast as you can, the bus carries on past you at 30 mph and the two scumbags get off at the next stop and intercept you.

b.   After where you live

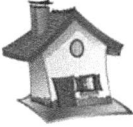

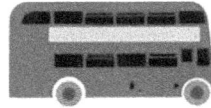

you live here

Direction of travel of the bus

Correct: you get off after where you live, start running as fast as you can, the bus carries on past you at 30 mph and the two scumbags get off at the next stop, but due to the buses speed you are already at least 500 metres in front of them. You arrive home safely!

I know it's not rocket science but you would not believe the amount of people who just do not know this simple stuff.

The same philosophy apply to trains, where to sit, near the driver. Again, you would be surprised how many people think that the driver sits at the rear of the train, bit difficult if he wants to see where he is going!

Sex

Men and women interpret sexual signals differently! Men are more likely to attribute sexual meaning to what women consider mere friendly behaviour. You have all probably heard the phrase "she was asking for it" or "she was gagging for it".

NO WOMAN EVER DESERVES TO BE RAPED!!!!!!!!!!!!!!!!!!!!

You could be walking down the street stark naked if you liked and you still would not deserve to be raped. You would not be doing yourself any favours by doing so, but the fact remains the same.

One typical way that men and women read sexual signals differently is;

If a good looking guy asked a girl out on a date, would the girl think there was anything wrong with that? Probably not. However,

If a girl asked a guy out on a date, what would the guy think?…….
whey hey…SEX.

I am not saying that you should be dressed in black bin liners when you go out, but you must realise that if you are "scantily clad" you will attract a certain amount of attention. If its 7 pm on a Friday evening and someone sees you not wearing much, they may wolf whistle you or shout complimentary things at you.

5 hours later when alcohol has been flowing freely, "Dutch courage" takes over and the guy may think he can get away with much more than a simple compliment.

This is why most guys will ask women out when they have been drinking. If you ask any guy about being embarrassed, they will tell you that there is nothing worse than being rejected by a girl.

What follows is again common sense, please don't think you are thick or plain daft if you don't know some of this information, in today's society we rely on automated things more and more, and we are losing the art of thinking for ourselves, therefore our minds become lazy.

Emergency phone numbers

We all know that the British emergency phone number is 999, and that USA emergency phone number is 911. How many people know that the emergency phone number for Europe is 112? If you go to Europe this is the only number that works, it works in the UK so I would get used to dialling this one just to be on the safe side.

If in doubt always call 999/112. The police would prefer you to call them and for you to have misunderstood the situation, rather than not calling them and finding you dead in a ditch somewhere!

<u>Mobile phones</u>

Can you dial the emergency services when you have no credit on your phone?

YES

Can you dial the emergency services when your key pad is locked?

YES

Can you dial the emergency services when you battery is dead?

OBVIUOSLY NOT

Can you use your mobile phone as weapon?

YES

Can you use your mobile phone to collect evidence, (photos, videos etc)

YES

<u>Cars</u>

Always keep your doors locked if you are travelling alone, traffic light muggings are on the increase.

If parking at night always ensure the area is well lit.

If parking in a multi storey car park, try to park as close as possible to the attendant's office.

If you breakdown on a motorway, put your hazard warning lights on, call the SOS box on the hard shoulder (even if you have your mobile phone on you, the boxes are tracked), they are free of charge and will put you in touch with the police.

Wait on the embankment of the road, not in your car, get out of the car via the passenger door, not the drivers door.

Always expect the unexpected.

<u>Personal Alarms</u>

This small gadgets are priceless when used in the correct situation. They vary in shape, design and indeed cost, but they all serve the same purpose and generally work the same way. They normally have a string attached to one end, which when pulled detaches itself from the main body, this then lets out a high pitched noise to attract attention. The only way this noise will stop is

a. If the string is put back in

b. If the battery dies

c. If it is stamped on or broken

As mentioned earlier do not expect help from any passer by, but to have a personal alarm is always advisable, you never know, some hero may come to your aid.

Do not rely on these too heavily, they are used as a distraction to help you run away. They are of no use if you are alone with your attacker, no one will hear the siren, but they are extremely effective in a densely populated area.

<u>Weapons</u>

There are an endless number of weapons that we can find in everyday objects, but it depends how and where to use them. The following list comes with the circumstances of when to use and how to use.

N.B. Pepper sprays and CS gas are illegal in the UK and you will face serious consequences if they are found in your possession. There are other things you could use:

Keys

Keys make a wonderful weapon but you have to be careful how and when you use them.

Remember

The Law:

"Section 3 of the Criminal Law Act 1967 states that a person may use force that is reasonable and necessary in the circumstance." It also states *"such a person must be able to justify their actions in a court of law"*

If you were just about to put your keys into your door after enjoying a night out and a stranger put their hand on your shoulder from behind (both you know and the attacker knows what his intentions are), you then turn around startled and gouge his eyes out with your keys. This is a serious incident and it would go to court.

What would you say when asked by the judge or the scumbags solicitor "why did you gouge this poor mans eyes out with your keys?"

What would be your response?

"The guy came from no where and attacked me from behind so I hit him with my keys"

Wrong answer, the man did not attack you, he merely put his hand on your shoulder. By giving the above answer you are saying that you intentionally used your keys as a weapon, you may go to prison.

The correct response would be

"I felt a hand on my shoulder whilst I was opening my door, it really startled me and I turned around to push the guy away from me, I totally forgot that my keys were in my hand."

All too often we see criminals getting off "scott free" and the victim is left injured and traumatised. I am not saying you should go around playing vigilante, but every human being has the fundamental right to defend themselves with the up most force, if that results in the attacker being injured or worse, then they only have themselves to blame.

On the other hand you couldn't use your keys if you were followed in a street far from where you lived with no cars present, and a guy put his hand on your shoulder in a bid to attack you.

If you did gouge his eyes out, what would you say in a court of law, why did you have your keys in your hand at the time of the attack?

There are other things you could use!

Hair brushes

There two types of hair brush available today.

One with steel bristles – hold the handle and swipe it about the attackers face

One with nylon bristles – hold the bristles and use the handle as a dagger

Any type of aerosol

This can include hairsprays, deodorants, antiperspirants, perfumes etc.

Spray into the eyes in order to escape

Lipstick

Most women these days, including my wife and daughter, use lip gloss instead of lip stick, lipsticks can prove to be a formidable weapon. Remove the top, keep the lip stick itself retracted and jab that into the attacker's cheek. The alloy is really soft and may break off in his face causing considerable pain.

Shoes

High heeled shoes can be taken off and used, or they can be left on the feet and used in a stamping motion straight through the attackers foot, straight into the concrete, (maybe in a grab from behind for example)

Mobile phones

As mentioned earlier

Credit cards

These have a really sharp edge to them, so maybe a swipe down the face may be used, but beware, you must be able to justify your actions. Why did you have your credit card in your hand at the time of the attack? There must be either an ATM or a bank nearby.

Finger rings

Turn the ring so that the stone is facing to the palm, so that if you slap your attacker the ring scratches his face. Who can say that your ring didn't slip around your finger during the attack.

Pens, pencils

Self explanatory

Books/magazines

When rolled up tight they can be used as batons, the edges really hurt

Handbags

Dependant upon size of course

The list goes on.

It has been in illegal since year 2000 to harass someone (Harassment Act 2000). In other words men cannot follow women for ages, tap them on their shoulder scaring them half to death, and then simply ask them for the time. If you are a victim of this type of assault report it as soon as possible.

It has also been generally known that you cannot use a pre-emptive strike (cannot hit first). RUBBISH! When I was growing up it was said that if you practiced a martial art, whether it be karate, judo, Tai Kwon Do etc., and you were threatened, you had to warn the attacker 3 times that you were a martial artist. What a load of CRAP! By the time you have finished your 3rd warning the attacker has either punched you, or at best is alerted to the fact that he may have to fight even dirtier to beat you.

When faced with a threatening situation, and you feel that your life may be in danger, you have every right to hit first and run, remember though, not hit, hit, hit, hit, hit, hit until he stops moving and then run.

The Law:

*"Section 3 of the Criminal Law Act 1967 states that **a person may use force that is reasonable and necessary in the circumstance.**"* It also states *"such a person must be able to justify their actions in a court of law"*

It is also a myth that you have to be really musically, or fit to deliver a powerful strike.

"Force = mass x acceleration"

If you hit with speed, you will create the force required to be able to escape.

Chapter 5
Chokes & Strangles

Chokes and strangles can be one of the most frightening things that you will encounter.

Extreme caution must be taken when practicing these techniques as accidents are bound to happen, especially when you begin to practice them at full speed.

Contrary to the British SAS, and the US navy seals who say it take 2 minutes to be put unconscious with a choke or strangle, trust me they are wrong. 7-10 seconds is the correct length of time, why? Because I have been choked personally and that is how long it took for me to be rendered unconscious.

The first thing that happens when you are choked or strangled is massive adrenalin dump (please refer to the information in "**Becoming Streetwise**")

After 3-4 seconds you will feel really nauseous, sick and in a state of shock.

After 7- 8 seconds you will start to black out.

After 10 seconds..............game over.

Whether we are being choked or strangle, whatever we do we must do it fast. In self defence we work on what is commonly know as the "3 S`s.

Strategy

Speed

Surprise

Strategy – always try to have a plan in place to deal with any form of attack

Speed – whatever you do, you must do it quickly, otherwise the assailant may read your moves and counter them

Surprise – the surprise part is the fact that you are fighting back. The attacker didn't expect this, after all he chose you because he thought you were going to be an easy target.

What is the difference between a choke and a strangle? A choke is from the back using the forearm of crease in the elbow, whilst a strangle is from the front using the hands.

Human nature commands both the same reflexes in both a choke and a strangle. As soon as someone puts their arm or hands around your neck, you raise your arms up to try pull the attacker off. This is the last thing you should do. Do you really think that he will let go of you if you do this?..........NO.. what will he do instead?, yep you guessed it, he will squeeze even tighter. Remember you only have 7-10 seconds to escape before you end up unconscious, by doing this silly but natural movement you are wasting valuable seconds.

Also remember what we also said at the beginning of this course. Every human being has 5 basic weapons, 2 arms, 2 legs, 1 head. Your attacker has already used 2 of his by choking you, you still have all your 5 left, don't waste them.

Chokes

A choke may be either standing choke, or a choke where you may be dragged backwards. Either way the results are the same, the forearm is pushed against the trachea and starves the lungs and brain of oxygen. A choke is the most dangerous form of attack....................you will not see it coming, one minute you are stood up, the next minute you're flat on your back. To briefly explain the 2 different types of arm position when ʿ ˡ ˙

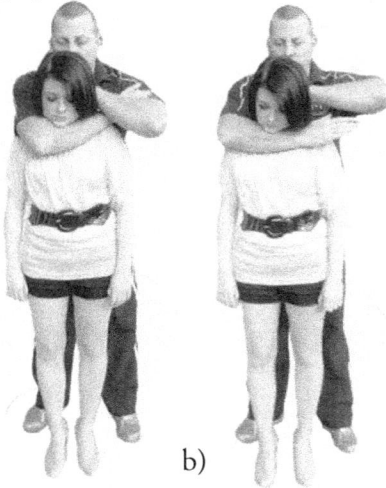

a)   b)

a.   The "sleeper".

This is when the assailant puts his arm across your throat and positions the crease of his elbow against your windpipe. He puts his other hand at the back of your head, locks the choking arm onto his other arm and begins to squeeze. At the same time his arm around your throat constricts, his bicep muscle and his forearm muscle are being tightened which in turn reduces the gap in the crease of his elbow, thus crushing your trachea.

b.   Ordinary choke.

This is nearly the same as above except the attackers arm is place straight across your windpipe and the actual forearm does the choking.

Results are exactly the same.

<u>To escape from a standing back choke</u>

DO NOT TRY TO PULL THE ATTACKERS ARMS OFF WITH YOUR ARMS, YOU

ARE SIMPLY WAST

ING TIME, REMEMBER YOU ONLY HAVE 7-10 SECONDS TO ESCAPE

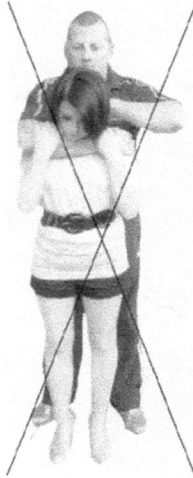

There is only one method of escaping this type of attack. Imagine the attacker has you in his grasp. We call this the 5 point plan, one of these movements will not work on their own, but putting them all together will work every time.

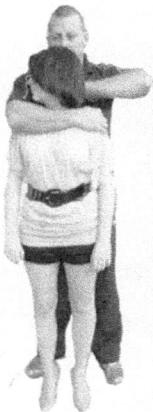 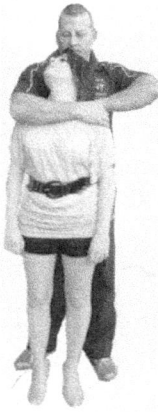 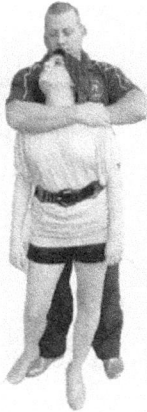 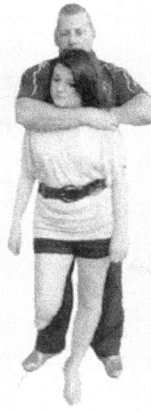 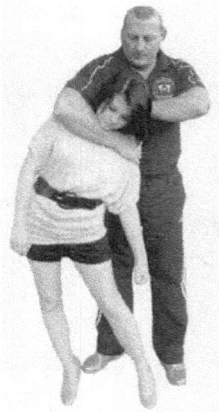

i)   ii)   iii)   iv)   v)

i. move your head towards toward his choking arms elbow so that your trachea is in the soft part of his elbow, this will buy you another couple of seconds of oxygen

ii. thrust your head straight back into his face, remember he is stood directly behind you, you will either break his nose or his chin. If the attacker is really tall, you will hit his sternum which is also very painful

iii. stamp as hard as possible onto his foot driving your shoe heal through his foot into the concrete, don't worry if you miss, have another go

iv. kick your heal backwards into his shins, if you miss, try again

v. lastly, keep your feet in the same position, but move your hips towards his choking arms elbow, keep your arm **straight** and swing it like a pendulum into his groin. By keeping the arm straight you have increased the surface area of your weapon

<u>To escape from a choke when you are being dragged backwards</u>

There are 2 very effective methods of escaping from this form of attack. We will tackle the easy one first, but before we do, do you agree with me that if you are attacked and pulled backwards, you are going to finish on the floor – yep that's exactly where the attacker wants you, either to rape you or rob you. With this in mind why not make it your idea to end up on the floor, if you are going to go down you might as well do it on your terms.

Method 1

When the attacker starts dragging you backwards simply hook one of your feet around one of his legs and he will inevitably fall over. Human nature says that he will probably let go of you to break his own fall, but hey if he doesn't, you don't care either way. You will land on top of him, with your head driving into his face totally destroying his ugly mush. Job Done!

Method 2

This is a little more complex, so please be patient while I break it down. As soon as the attacker begins to drag you backwards turn your whole body towards the fingers of his choking arm and drop immediately to your knees. (Yes you will probably graze or cut your knees, but that's not half as much as you are going to do to your assailant). Once on your knees you will find that your head is facing his groin, do not bite, you do not know what he has got. Grab anything that comes to hand, tear, squeeze, rip, twist. I guarantee you he will let go. Then put one arm around his legs, joined by your other arm and perform a rugby tackle as he continues to walk backwards. As before, human nature states that he will let go of your neck so that he may break his own fall. This may not be the most graceful technique but it works every time. Once he is flat on the floor, hit his groin and run.

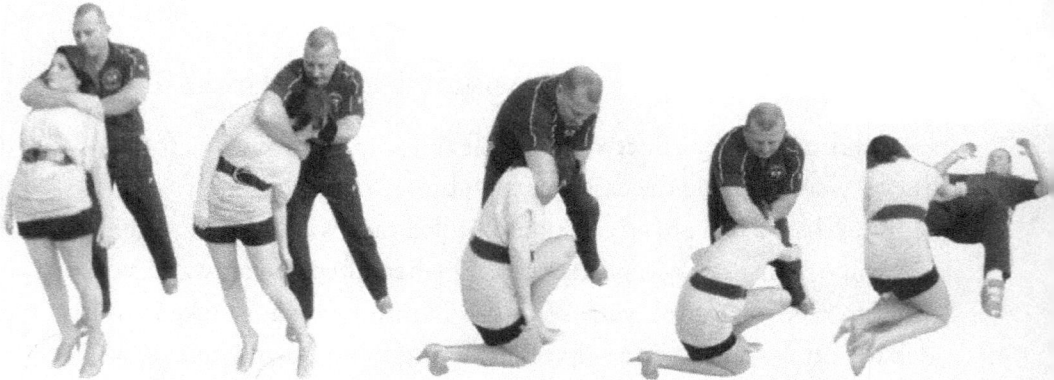

Strangles

Strangles are less dangerous than a choke in that you can see the attack coming. It is more dangerous in the respect that when the hands are about the throat, the thumbs crush the trachea from behind whilst the fingers squeeze the carotid artery and jugular veins at the side of the neck. So as well as starving your lungs of oxygen, your brain will also be starved of blood.

If someone manages to get their hands around your throat, your fist instinct is a good one, kick them straight in the groin. If they see this coming and turn their body sideways there are still other ways to escape. Some take years of practice to perfect and some do not work if the guy is excessively strong, so we have kept these techniques simple. I personally have done the "guillotine" on a 24 stone man who was strangling me (he did not believe that it would work), bearing in mind I weigh in at only 13 stone, he was more than a little amazed when I nearly broke his wrists.

Method 1

Bring your hands up in between his arms (don't go around the outside as he may read this action and put you in an arm lock) and poke his eyes out. His body action will make him pull his head away from you and at the same time push his groin toward you. I don't have tell you what to do next.

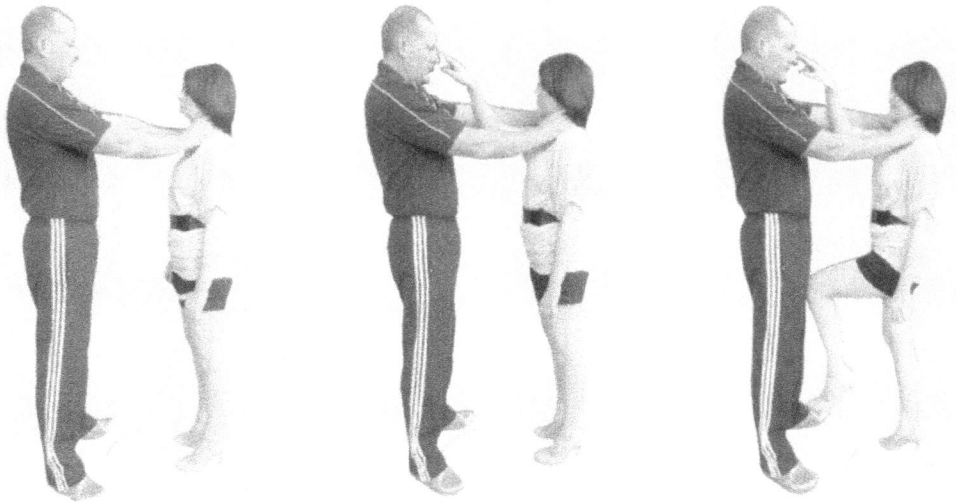

Method 2

The "Guillotine". Every human body has weak points, even if they are body builders or really fit people go for the joints, joints are one of the weakest parts of body. If the guy has you in strangle, lift one arm vertically into the air, then take a large step back with the opposite leg. You must now turn 180° so you are facing away from attacker bringing your vertical arm down simultaneously so that the palm of your hand slaps your opposite hip (the hip of the leg that you have stepped back with). This will render your attacker off balance coming towards you, you have his hands trapped under your guillotine arm and his wrists have broken, then while he is still falling towards you, drive the same guillotine arms elbow straight into his face. You walk off smiling, he is laying on the floor. Good night!

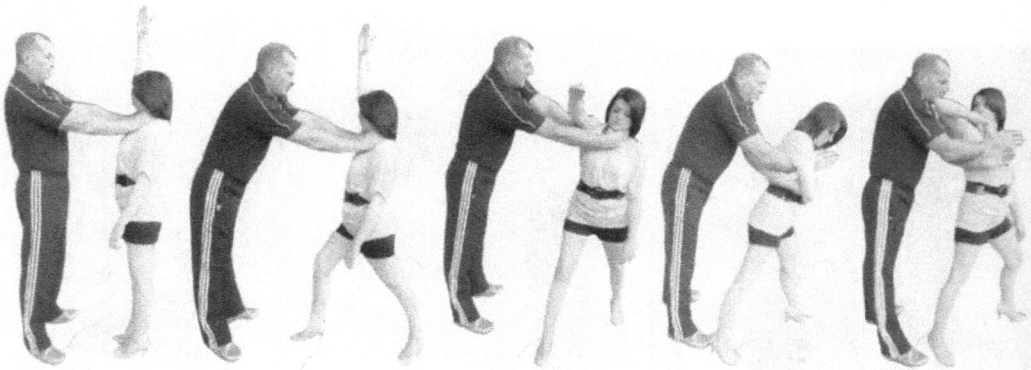

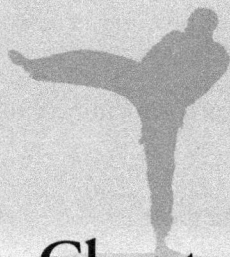

Chapter 6
Knives and guns

I have tried to keep this chapter to a minimum, the reason being is that I could spend pages and pages trying to teach you knife defences and gun defences. I have read countless books and watched endless DVD`s / recordings on YouTube, from ex forces people who are "experts" in this field. All look very impressive, but in real life when adrenaline takes over and the threat of a knife attack is imminent, trust me, you will not remember a thing. The average person has not spent years in the special-forces conducting "black Ops" behind enemy line, the fact of the matter is this;

I have been working with knives for over 25 years and if I were attacked I would get cut, slashed and stabbed. The knife defences that we teach our karate students are taken from the Israeli martial art of Krav Maga (a brutal but effective system used by the Israeli armed forces). They are designed to save your life, they will not stop you getting cut. The last thing I would want, is for you to think you know how to defend against a knife, get involved in an incident and instead of running away, you try to practice the techniques and end up DEAD.

One really important rule is – if an attacker wants your money or valuables – give it to them.

They would typically hold the knife in one hand and hold their other hand palm upwards waiting for you to hand over your valuables. DO NOT place your valuables in their hand. Throw your goods at him under arm (non threatening way) and aim for his knees, the goods will fall to the floor and his reaction will be to bend down and pick them up.

At this stage run, do not go toward him and try to knee him in his head, remember he still has the knife.

The question I get asked the most is;

"What if he robs me, then stabs me?"

The chances of this happening are really slim. The attacker is using the weapon as a threat, nothing more. Think about it, if the guy wanted you dead he would kill you and then rob you, he still has your possessions.

If in doubt RUN!

If running is not an option and an attack is certain, by all means use all methods at your disposal. Please refer to phrase at the beginning of this book, "prevention is better than the cure", not being in the wrong place at the wrong time. Obviously there are always exceptions to the rule but we are talking about minimising your risk of attack.

For more information regarding weapon defences, please seek professional tuition from a fully qualified instructor. Hands on practice is far better than book reading or DVD watching, but I will say this again.........

"When adrenaline takes over and the threat of a knife attack is imminent, trust me, you will not remember a thing."

Chapter 7
Grabs & Holds

In this chapter we shall try to educate in the different forms of grabs, holds, and locks.

Wrist hold

Someone is holding your wrist tight as a restraining technique and you cannot get away. The first thing is to trust your instincts and kick him in groin. If he reads this and turns to the side, then there are still things you can do?

There are two ways someone may grab your wrist, either same side, or opposites. What I mean by this is;

Same side – in that the person is holding your right wrist for example with their left hand, same side of your bodies

Opposite side – in that the person is holding your right wrist for example with their own right wrist, opposite side of your bodies.

The technique for escape is the same. As mentioned before joints are the weakest parts of the body regardless of strength, fingers and thumbs are no different. We must move towards thumbs, fingers are brilliant things in that they perform all types of functions.

Thumbs however are limited to holding or gripping functions. For example try to grab someone using just your fingers and not your thumbs, your victim can escape relatively easily.

If someone grabs your wrist your initial reaction is to pull away, if they grab your forearm and you pull, their grip will simply slide down to your wrist and stay there. Fists are wider that wrists.

Plan A: We must use large circles to escape from such attacks.

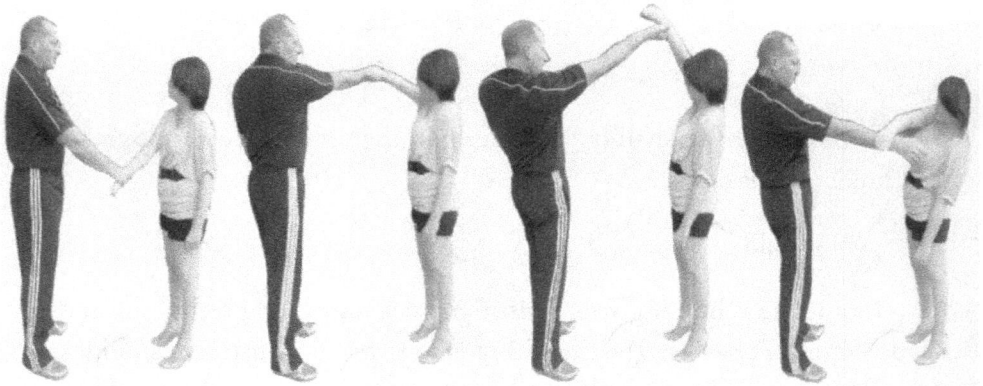

Once someone has grabbed your wrist you must use psychology. I have had numerous instances where I have taught this technique and the woman has tried it on their partners and obviously the man wants to prove a point so they grab really tight and use all their upper body strength to keep a grip. The woman then tells me it is rubbish and doesn't work. I feel angry because I know these systems work. Human nature states that if you pull one way then the attacker will pull the other way to neutralise your power.

At the beginning of this course I said that 70% of self defence is mental awareness. So here is what you do;

When the strong macho man grabs your wrist, start to push toward the fingers (I know this is the opposite of which you should be moving, but please bear with me.). Human nature dictates that the man will try and resist you, excellent, once you are confident he is giving it his all, simply pull toward the thumb in a large circular motion. At the same time as you do this kick his shins really hard......he will let go....and probably swear at you.

Plan B: Simply "rap" the back of the guys hand with your knuckles.... he will let go !

What happens if the man grabs both your wrists so that they are positioned upwards with your elbows pointing vertically downwards? Same rules as before........pull away to the outside, the assailant will instantly resist and push back trying to close you arms so that your forearms will be touching, you then open your palms, like a flower opens its petals.

This will expose his thumbs as he grips you, use his force combined with your force and smash his thumbs together, ouch!

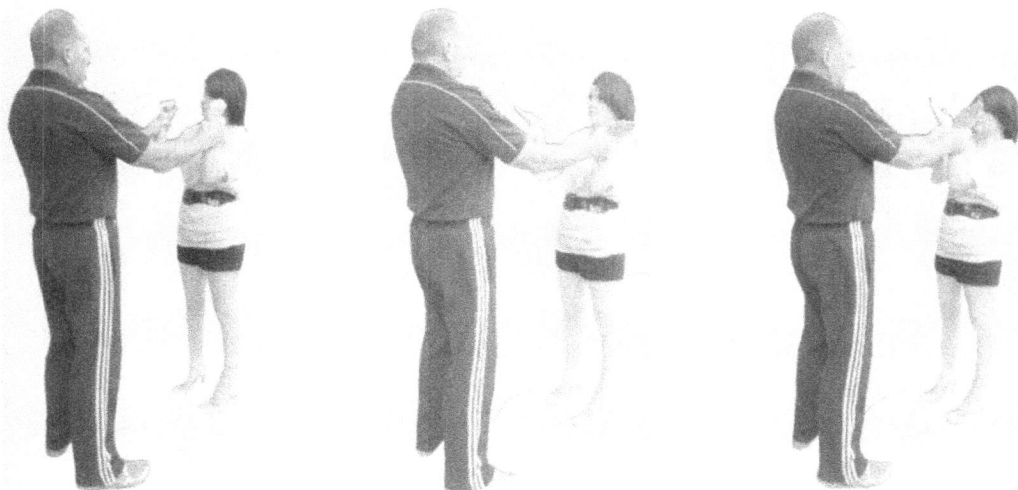

<u>Lapel grab</u>

Imagine someone grabbing your lapels, could be a man or even another woman, what is on their mind. Yep, they want to head butt you. As usual we try to keep this stuff simple. As he pulls you toward him, raise one of your arms up through the middle of his arms (as explained in strangles, not going around the outside) with your index finger and forefinger slightly spread, that's it just leave them in that position. The attacker's momentum of pulling you toward him, he will ultimately poke himself in the eyes, but with your fingers.

Alternatively use the "guillotine" method as described in strangles in the previous chapter.

<u>Grabs from behind</u>

There are two types of grab from behind:

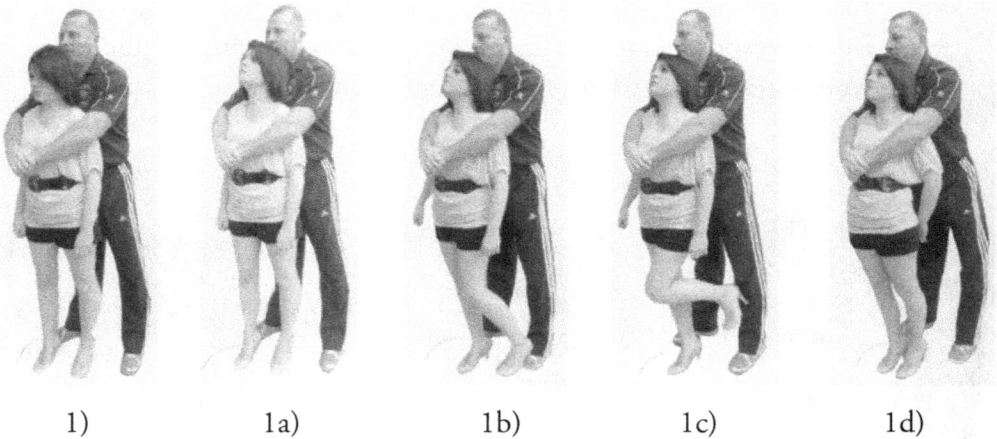

1)   1a)   1b)   1c)   1d)

1.   The attacker comes up behind you, places his arms over the tops of your arms nearyour shoulders and squeezes, general "bear hug" position. Remember your weapons,you still have 5 left. So in a similar way to being choked;

a.   thrust your head straight back into his face, remember he is stood directly behind you, you will either break his nose or his chin. If the attacker is really tall, you will hit his sternum which is also very painful

b.   stomp as hard as possible onto his foot driving your shoe heal through his foot into the concrete, don't worry if you miss, have another go

c.   kick your heal backwards into his shins, again if you miss, try again

d.   reach behind you and grab and squeeze whatever comes to hand!

2.   The attacker come up behind you, puts his arms under yours and squeezes, similar to the "Heimlich Manoeuvre". As before do every thing, a,b,c and d, if he still doesn't let go, "play Tarzan" on his hands. You know the thing when Tarzan cried out to bring all the animals to his rescue whilst at the same time beating his chest. That's exactly what you must do, sure shout of if you want, but instead of beating your chest, rap the backs of his hands with your fists, he will soon let go!

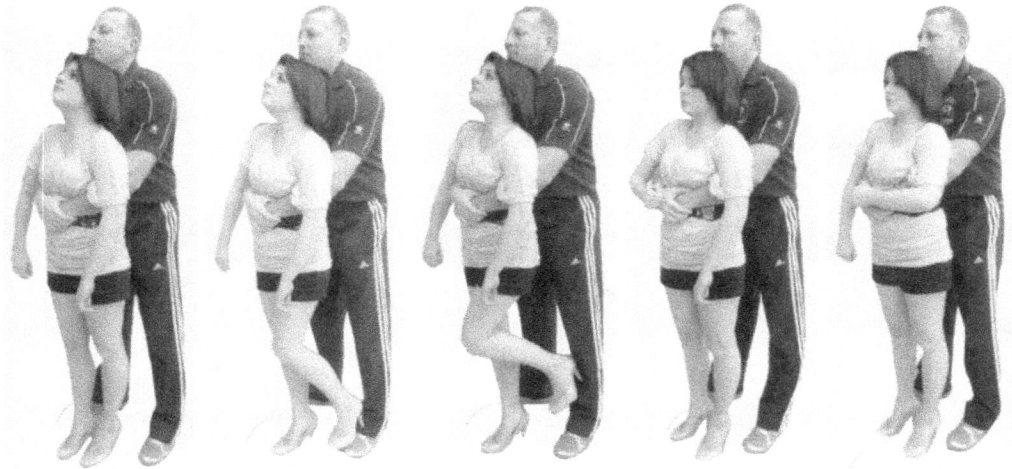

Grabs from the front

There are two types of grab from the front, as above the arms come either over or under the arms:

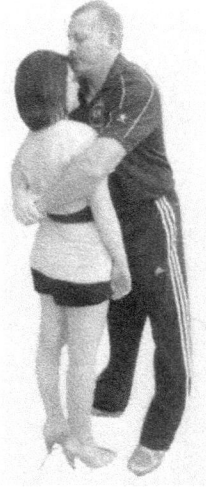 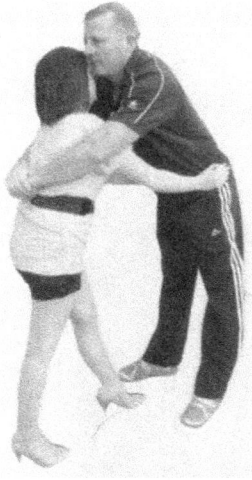 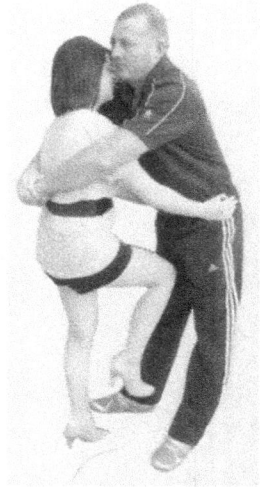

1)   1a)   1b)

1.   The attacker comes up to you, places his arms over the top of your arms near your shoulders and squeezes, general "bear hug position". Remember your weapons, you still have 5 left, although you cannot get your hands up to his face.

a.   place your hands on the attackers hips, step backwards with one leg and push away.

b.   this will create enough space for you to knee him in his groin.

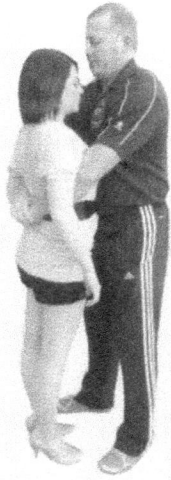 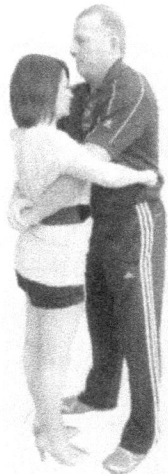 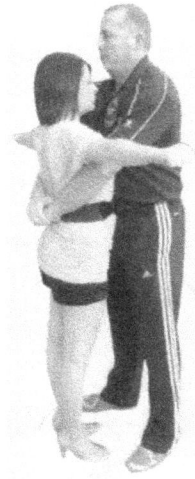

2)   2a)   2b)

2.   The attacker comes up to you, places his arms under your arms and squeezes.

a.   use your finger to get to his eyes, use the heal of your hand thrusting upwards into his septum of his nose, put your fingers and thumb around his windpipe and turn 90 °, cup your hands to his ears bursting his ear drums, punch his nose, his chin (all head atemi wazas as discussed earlier)

b.   after this make a normal fist but with your thumbs resting on the top of the fist, this makes a pointed object, slam both fists in to the attackers floating ribs (this area can easily be found, if run your fingers down the side seam of you're shirt until you come to "fleshy bit" of your side – you've found it). It tickles when pushed but wow does it hurt when punched.

Hair grabs

Most women have long hair and tie them up in pony tails, although this may look very pretty, it also gives a potential attacker a natural leverage on which to hurt you. Hair grabs are usually done from behind, but even from the front, the same principles apply.

Your instinct when having your hair pulled is to pull away, try not to do this as you may lose your hair! The attacker will probably be stood quite a distance away from you (unlike a back choke) so the techniques such as shi kicking or stamping on insteps may not work. Not to worry, here is what you do;

As the attacker has grabbed your hair he automatically makes a fist. Don't panic. Place one of you hands on top of his fist and press down really hard onto your own skull, put your other hand on top of this one and push again. This will give you a headache, but that's nothing compared to what you will do to him.

Once you have secured his fist by pressing all your fingers into the crevices of his fist, begin to turn 180° toward your attacker bending at the knee as you do so. Start to walk him backwards, DO NOT LET GO OF HIS FIST, with your hands still glued to your head, while his wrists, elbows and shoulders are being either broken or dislocated, knee his groin and run..........happy days!

NB, the lower you bend when turning, the more pressure you will exert on to his joints.

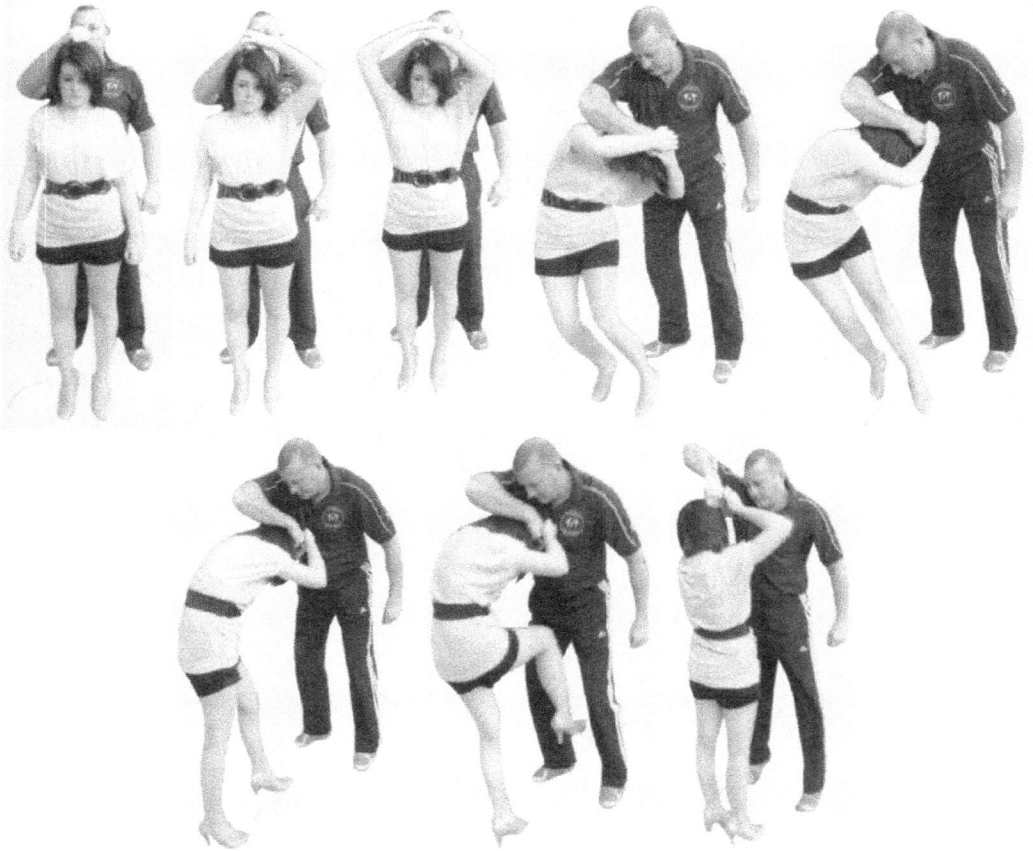

Chapter 8
Basic 1st Aid

All professional martial artists must be 1st aid trained, I am no different. Obviously 1st aid is a huge subject and I could fill a whole book just on this subject alone. The following bullet points will hopefully help you, if you either come across someone in distress, or you, God forbid, are a victim yourself.

The main phrase that we use in 1st aid is:

DRAB

D = Danger

You must ensure the site is safe before you go to work on a patient. There is not much point giving CPR (cardiopulmonary resuscitation) to a road traffic accident casualty if you are going to be knocked over by oncoming traffic. Make sure nothing can fall on you, ladders etc, make sure electrical cables are clear and isolated.

R = Response

How do you know if the person is not just sleeping? We need to get a response. Start by talking to them ("are you ok mate" or something similar), slightly shaking them on the shoulders, nipping the casualties skin either on their face or inside the upper arm. If there is still no response we know something is wrong.

A = Airway

The primary cause of death is suffocation or the inability to breath, without oxygenated air the brain dies in 3-4 minutes, without the brain the rest of the body is useless. Very rarely do victims collapse in the flat laid down position, normally they are a crumpled heap. If they are not flat, be careful how you move them, you never know the casualty could have a neck injury. Once flat, we can begin to check the airway. It is a myth that you can swallow your tongue, it merely falls back and covers the trachea. If you suspect the casualty has a neck injury you must perform "a jaw thrust" to open the mouth. If not, put a heel of the hand on the forehead, the other hand on the chin and push the forehead backwards. This opens the mouth, remove any object carefully, tongue, food, chewing gum etc, and carry on checking for breathing. We do this by letting go of the head, placing our cheek over the casualty's mouth and nose and look downwards towards the casualty's feet. If the person is breathing we shall see his chest cavity rising and falling.

If all checks out we must put the casualty into the recovery position

B = Bleeding

The secondary cause of death is bleeding to death. Looking for severe blood loss and stopping it can be critical to the survival of the casualty.

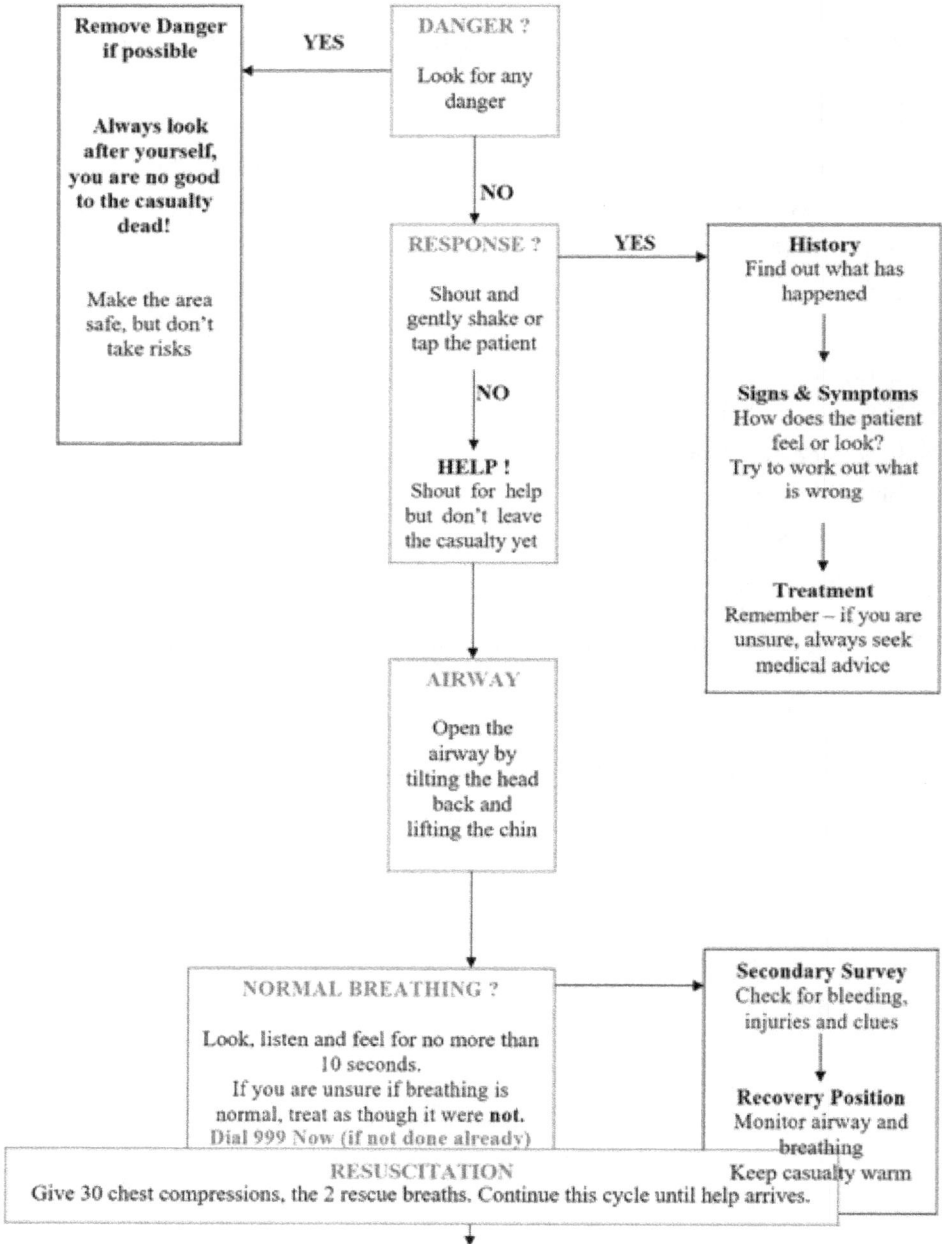

Dial 999

	DANGER ?		
Remove Danger if possible ← YES —	Look for any danger		

Remove Danger if possible

Always look after yourself, you are no good to the casualty dead!

Make the area safe, but don't take risks

↓ **NO**

RESPONSE ? — YES →

Shout and gently shake or tap the patient

↓ **NO**

HELP !
Shout for help but don't leave the casualty yet

History
Find out what has happened

↓

Signs & Symptoms
How does the patient feel or look?
Try to work out what is wrong

↓

Treatment
Remember – if you are unsure, always seek medical advice

AIRWAY

Open the airway by tilting the head back and lifting the chin

NORMAL BREATHING ? →

Look, listen and feel for no more than 10 seconds.
If you are unsure if breathing is normal, treat as though it were **not**.
Dial 999 Now (if not done already)

Secondary Survey
Check for bleeding, injuries and clues

↓

Recovery Position
Monitor airway and breathing
Keep casualty warm

RESUSCITATION
Give 30 chest compressions, the 2 rescue breaths. Continue this cycle until help arrives.

Cardiac compressions should be done with the heal of the hand in the middle of the chest (approximately between the nipples). On adults and adolescents interlock the fingers and with arms straight push downwards. N.B. not enough pressure will do nothing to massage the heart. On babies and young children use two fingers to push.

Dependant upon the size and age of the casualty use either, 2 hands, 1 hand or 2 fingers to push.

The rate of these cardiac compressions is one per second....... "1 and 2 and 3 and 4 and 5 and so on.

Some people may feel uncomfortable about giving mouth to mouth resuscitation. If you have no mouth guard and think your life may be at risk, then doing the cardiac compressions only is an option. Doing something is better than doing nothing. A rate of 100 compressions per minute should be maintained.

It is common for a person who has stopped breathing to vomit whilst unconscious. This is a passive action so you may not see or hear it happening. You might not find out until you give a rescue breath, (as the air comes back out of the patient it will make a gurgling sound)

If the patient has vomited, turn them onto their side, tip the head back and allow the vomit to run out.

Clean the face of the patient and continue with resuscitation using a protective face guard if possible.

As said before, always look after No1.

- wipe the patients lips clean

- use a mouth guard like "resuci-aid" if possible

- if not use a plastic bag with a hole in it, or even a handkerchief

- wear protective gloves

The recovery position is easy when you know how, (although there are many forms of the recovery position the one shown below is, we believe, the easiest one to perform:

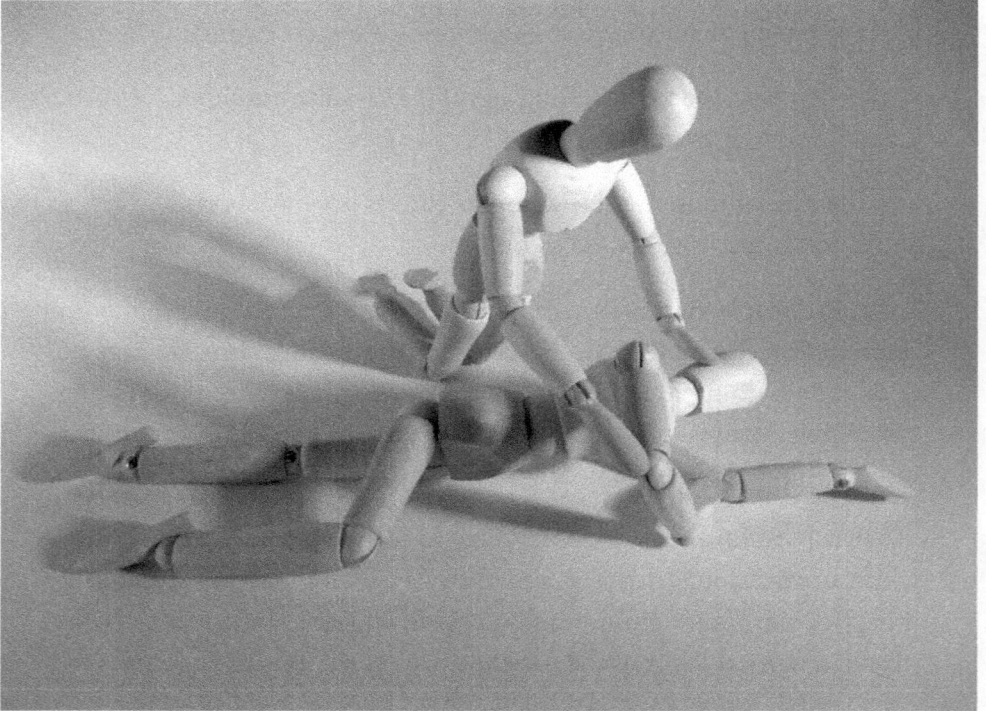

One of the main rules in 1ˢᵗ aid is the "BBB" rule. If you should come across a multi casualty incident how do you decide who needs treatment first?, use BBB. Always care for the quite ones first. If they are quite it is probable that they are not breathing, if they are noisy and screaming out in pain at least you know that they are alive.

B = Breathing, ensure the casualty is breathing, if they can't breathe they die!

B = Bleeding, try to stem major blood loss

B = Bones

Choking

If a person is choking, firstly encourage the person to cough. If it is not serious this may do the trick. If the obstruction is not cleared:

Back slaps – bend the casualty over so the head is below the chest. Give 5 firm blows between the shoulder blades with the palm of your hand. Check between blows and stop if you clear the obstruction

Abdominal thrusts – stand behind the casualty, place both your arms around their waist. Make a fist with one hand and place it over the abdomen, below the ribs with your thumb inwards. Grasp the fist with your other hand and pull sharply inwards and upwards. Do this 5 times checking between thrusts, stop if you are successful.

Repeat the above steps, ask some one to dial 999 fro an ambulance just in case.

If the patient becomes unconscious, support the casualty to the ground and begin CPR.

Warning. Abdominal thrusts can cause serious internal injuries, always send the patient to see a doctor.

Choking on a child can be just as dangerous. Use the same techniques as above but use common sense when determining how much strength is to be used.

Abdominal thrusts should not be performed on a baby.

Bleeding

Bleeding can come from many sources, capillaries, arteries, veins etc. What is the difference? Capillaries may probably stop themselves. Arteries are extremely frightening, they follow the same rhythm as the heart, and so every time that the heart pumps, so does the artery. This is why sometimes blood could spurt out over a considerable distance. Veins tend to bleed more steadily, but they are just as dangerous.

If someone is bleeding heavily use **S.E.E.P.**

Sit or lay – the casualty down in a comfortable but appropriate position to the wound

Examine – look for foreign objects and note how it is bleeding (vein or artery)

Elevate – ensure the wound is above the level of the heart, use gravity to reduce blood flow

Pressure – apply pressure to stem the bleeding, if an object is present, press either side.

If there is an object in the wound, DO NOT remove, simply apply sterile dressing around it.

"Tourniquets" are a controversial issue. They used to be common place in 1st aid, but if they were left on for too long gangrene set in and people would lose their limbs. My advice is again based on common sense. If a casualty is bleeding really heavily with a major arterial injury for example and blood is going everywhere. You may have only 2 choices;

a.   Let the person bleed to death or

b.   Apply a tourniquet, but release every so often to decrease tissue damage.

Shock

Shock can be a major factor in fatalities. The definition of shock is "a lack of oxygen to the tissues of the body which is caused by a fall in blood volume or blood pressure"

Severe bleeding can result in shock, which can kill. An average adult caries around 10 pints of blood in their body, while a child only has 4 pints. So remember a child can "bleed out" much faster than an adult can.

The signs of someone in shock are

a.   Pale, clammy skin (with blue or grey tinges if it is severe)

b.   Dizziness or fainting (especially if they try to stand or sit up)

c.   Rapid, shallow breathing

Eye injuries

If a person gets dust or something really small in their eye, it can be washed out with cold tap water, ensure the flow runs away from the good eye.

If it is more serious, place a soft sterile dressing over both eyes to stop the injured eye from moving, eyes move in unison.

If a person gets chemicals in their eyes wash out with copious amounts of water, cover eyes with a soft sterile dressing and take to hospital. Under no circumstance should you wash out with salt or a saline solution. I know this from experience;

Some years ago when I had a "proper job" as my wife calls it, I accidentally got a chemical called aliphatic amine splashed in my eyes. My colleague (I did call him something else at the time) washed my eyes out with a saline solution form the 1st aid kit. This added to the injury and I was rushed to hospital, after undergoing tests etc, it was found that I had burnt the skin off both eyeballs and the saline had contributed to this. My wife had to literally apply the prescribed cream by the use of her fingers to my eyes – very painful.

SO PLEASE JUST USE CLEAN COLD TAP WATER!

Nose bleeds

DO NOT push the head back. Blood flows down the trachea and can either choke you or make you vomit (blood and hydrochloric acid in your stomach do not mix).

DO NOT nip the bridge of the nose, the casualty may have broken it, and he will definitely let you know if you hurt him.

Nip the soft part of the nose whilst tilting the head forward. Keep the pressure on for up to 10 minutes if required, telling the patient to breathe through his mouth. Advise the patient not to breathe through or blow their nose for a few hours after the bleeding has stopped.

If still bleeding, take to A & E.

<u>Burns</u>

There are 2 different types of burns, wet and dry.

Dry burns include things like fire, touching hot cookers etc

Wet or moist burns include things like scalding, steam etc.

The outcomes are exactly the same and the 1st aid is the same too.

• cool the burn under preferably running cold water for 10 minutes (if water is not available, use cold milk, pop etc.)

• remove jewellery and loosen clothing

• dress the burn

DO NOT

Burst blisters

Touch the burn

Apply lotions, ointments or fats

Apply adhesive tape or dressings

Remove clothing that has stuck to the burn

<u>Spinal injuries</u>

Again common sense to be used. Try not to move the casualty if a neck or spinal injury is suspected, however if the patient is choking on his own vomit, he will die anyway form lack of air. The worst scenario would be for a casualty to die though asphyxiation but when asked why you turn around and say "ah but look as his spine, it is as straight as you will ever see", the bloke is still dead though. You may think that is funny, but it really does happen.

If you come across someone in such a state

• reassure the patient, tell them not to move

• keep the patient in the position you find them

• hold their head still with your hands, keep the head and neck in line with the upper body.

• Dial 999 for an ambulance and keep the casualty still and warm until help arrives.

What if the patient is unconscious?

• If the casualty is breathing normally, this means that the airway must be clear so there is no need to tip the head backward. (you may have to perform a jaw thrust if they are not)

• Dial 999 for an ambulance

• Hold the head still with your hands, keep the neck and head in line with the upper body

• If you have to leave the casualty, if they begin to vomit, or if you are concerned about their airway, you should put them into the recovery position. Keep the head and neck in line with the spinal column while you turn them

• Keep the casualty warm and still, constantly monitor breathing until help arrives. Only move the patient if they are in severe danger.

Heart attack

Symptoms:

• Vice like pain in the centre of the chest (sometimes can be mistaken for indigestion)

• The pain can sometimes spread into either arm, the neck, jaw, back or shoulders

• Pale, cold clammy skin, going into shock

• Pulse variation

• Nausea or vomiting

• Severe sweating

• Shortness of breath

• Dizziness or weakness

Treatment of a heart attack

• sit the casualty down and make them comfortable. A half sitting position is best (the "W" position), this is where the patient is sat up against something with his legs bent at the knee and feet flat on the floor

• dail 999 for an ambulance

• if the patient suffers from angina, give them their medication to administer themselves

• reassure casualty

• monitor pulse and breathing

Stroke

There are 2 types of stroke,

A blood clot blocking a blood vessel supplying a part of the brain or

A blood vessel bursts and bleeds into the brain cavity, this puts pressure on the brain.

The outcome of a stroke depends entirely on which area and how much of the brain is affected

Signs and symptoms:

- weakness or paralysis down one side of the body or face

- slurred, confused or problems with speech

- gradual or sudden loss of consciousness

- agitation or aggression to the point of crying

- headache

- slow strong pulse

- slow deep, noisy breathing

- may have unequal pupil size

- flushed, dry skin

- vomiting or incontinence

Treatment of a stroke

- check airway and breathing

- dial 999 for an ambulance

- place *unconscious* casualty in the recovery position

- lay the *conscious* casualty down, with head and shoulders raised

- reassure casualty

- monitor and record breathing, pulse and consciousness

as seen on T.V.

- Facial weakness

- Arm weakness

- Speech problems

- Test these signs

Diabetes

Diabetes is a condition suffered by a person who does not produce enough insulin.

Insulin works in your blood stream to "burn of" the sugars that you eat. Some diabetic people have such a lack of insulin that they need to have insulin injections to keep their sugars down. An insulin diabetic has to make sure that they eat the correct amount of sugar to match the insulin they are injecting. If the balance is wrong they can go "hypo" or hypoglycaemic. If they don't eat enough sugar (missing a meal for example) the insulin injection with carry on burning off sugar left in the blood stream and their blood sugars become dangerously low.

Low blood sugar is dangerous because brain cells, unlike any other cells, can only use glucose as their energy supply, so the brain is literally starved.

In simple terms there must be a balance;

Too much insulin $\mathbf{V}$ too little sugar $=$ DANGER

Too little insulin $\mathbf{V}$ **too much sugar** $=$ DANGER

Sign and Symptoms

• bizarre, uncharacteristic, uncooperative, violent, sometimes mistaken for drunkenness

• confusion, memory loss

• may deteriorate into unconsciousness

• pale, cold sweaty skin

• shallow rapid breathing, fast pulse

• visual signs such as, the patient may wear a medic-alert bracelet, they may be carrying insulin, glucose tablets etc

Treatment of low blood sugar

• give the casualty a sugary drink, sugar lumps. Glucose tablets

• if they respond quickly, give them more food and drinks, stay with them until they get back to normal

• if they do not respond to treatment with 10 minutes, call 999 for an ambulance

• if the patient becomes unconscious maintain airway and breathing, place in the recovery position and wait until help arrives

<u>Fitting (also called seizures or convulsions)</u>

The majority of people who have this condition follow a pattern, they do things one step after the other. In this order;

• AURA – if they feel a fit coming on they will get to a safe place away from everyone

• TONIC – their body becomes stiff as all their muscles go into spasm, these will only last for around 30 seconds

• CLONIC – arms and legs start lashing about, eyes may roll backward, teeth clench, saliva may drool from the mouth (this may be red if the casualty has bit their own tongue). The patient may lose control of their bladder or bowel, this phase will last around 2 minutes

• RECOVERY – the casualty may go into a deep sleep or become really confused.

Treatment of fitting

During the fit -

• help the patient to the floor to avoid injury

• move dangerous objects away from the patient

• gently protect the head with a piece of clothing or your hands

• time the fit

• loosen any tight clothing around the neck

• dial 999 for an ambulance

After a fit –

• check airway and breathing

• place patient in the recovery position

- move bystanders away before they awake to protect modesty

- dial 999 for an ambulance

- constantly monitor airway and breathing

<u>Broken arms</u>

Reassure the casualty. If no slings are available, place the arm gently inside a shirt and take to hospital

<u>Dislocated shoulder</u>

Leave the casualty alone, reassure and take to hospital. DO NOT attempt to move the arm as the casualty will probably slap you for your troubles.

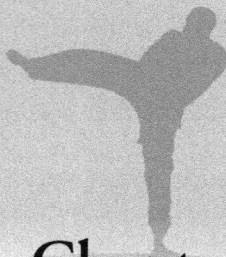

Chapter 9
Recap

As promised earlier please find below a short quiz, nothing major, just a bit of fun. The answers are on the next page in RED. The gaps in the sentences are answers, if there are 2 gaps, there are 2 answers. The numbers in brackets at the end of the question signifies how many points can be scored. Good luck!

QUIZ (33)

1. YOU CAN USE FORCE THAT IS .... AND .... IN THE CIRCUMSTANCE. (2)

2. CAN YOU .... YOUR ACTIONS? (1)

3. WHAT IS FIGHT OR FLIGHT RESPONSE? .... (1)

4. WHAT IS ADRENALINE DUMP? .... (1)

5. LEARN TO GET YOUR .... ON THE SAME LEVEL AS YOUR OPPONENTS .... (2)

6. IF YOU HAVE NO CREDIT ON YOUR PHONE AND IT IS LOCKED WHO CAN YOU STILL RING? ....(1)

7. IF YOU COME UP TO AN ALLEY WAY, WHAT SHOULD YOU DO? .... (1)

8. CAN YOU USE A PRE-EMPTIVE FIRST STRIKE? .... (1)

9. WHAT SHOULD YOU LOOK FOR IN A TAXI CAB?(2)
....

10. HOW LONG BEFORE A STANDING CHOKE OR STRANGLE PUTS YOU UNCONSCIOUS? .... (1)

11. IF AN ATTACKER HAS A BLADE AT YOUR THROAT, WHAT SHOULD YOU DO? ....(1)

12. IF AN ATTACKER WANTS YOUR MONEY OR VALUABLES, WHAT SHOULD YOU DO? .... (1)

13. WHAT EQUATION MAKES FOR A POWERFUL STRIKE? .... (1)

14. NAME 3 FENCES. .... (3)

15. HOW FAR TALKING DISTANCE?................................ (1)

16. NAME 3 OF THE BODIES MOST VULNERABLE POINTS .... (3)

17) IF AN ATTACKER GRABS YOU, SHOULD YOU TAKE THEIR ARMS OFF OR STRIKE FIRST? .... (1)

18. NAME 5 EVERYDAY THINGS YOU CAN USE AS A WEAPON .... (5)

19. WHAT PHONE NUMBER ABROAD GETS YOU THROUGH TO THE EMERGENCY SERVICES? .... (1)

20. a) WHAT YEAR DID THE CRIMINAL LAW ACT COME IN ....(1)

b) WHAT YEAR DID THE HARASSMENT ACT COME IN .... (1)

21) IF YOU ARE ATTACKED YOU MUST GO TO THE POLICE STATION TO REPORT IT, DO YOU: (1)

a) MAKE OUT A STATEMENT AS SOON AS POSSIBLE, OR

b) WAIT FOR SOLICITOR TO SPEAK TO YOU AND HELP YOU WITH THE STATEMENT

TOTAL:

ANSWERS

1. reasonable   necessary

2. justify

3. fight or run away

4. makes you freeze

5. reactions   actions

6. 999 / 112 / emergency services

7. cross over the road

8. yes

9. licence plate on the outside   I.D. badge on the inside

10. 7-10 seconds

11. nothing, stay absolutely still, do not move, he may accidentally cut you, give him what he wants

12. give him what he wants

13. force = mass x acceleration

14. staggered, submissive, psychological

15. arms length

16. eyes, throat, groin

17. strike first

18. keys, credit cards, hand bags, mobile phones, aerosols, pens, shoes, hair brushes, rings, etc

19. 112 for Europe, 999 for USA

20. a) 1967   b) 2000

21. b) wait for a solicitor to come

The main principles of self-defence are to lower the risk of you becoming a victim, keep your eyes open and your wits about you. Your fear will be over come by confidence. Hopefully you will never have to use the skills taught, but it is always better to be safe than sorry.

I hope I have not made you into a shaking paranoid lump of jelly after all this, but a little paranoia is good, it will heighten your awareness and help you to look for the danger signs early.

So please walk with confidence, trust your instincts and please STAY SAFE!

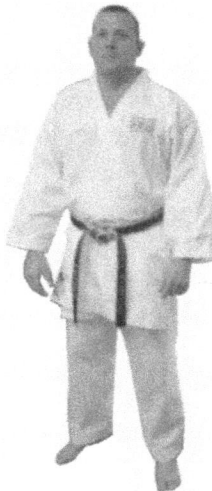

www.ingramcontent.com/pod-product-compliance
Lightning Source LLC
Chambersburg PA
CBHW032101020426

42335CB00011B/448